Review Questions for
MICROBIOLOGY
AND IMMUNOLOGY

A Review for the USMLE
Step 1, 2 and 3 Examinations

Review Questions for
MICROBIOLOGY
AND IMMUNOLOGY

A Review for the USMLE
Step 1, 2 and 3 Examinations

by

Andy C. Reese, PhD (Editor)
Cherukantath N. Nair, PhD
George H. Brownell, PhD

Department of Immunology and Microbiology
Medical College of Georgia

Review Questions Series
Series Editor: Thomas R. Gest, PhD
University of Arkansas for Medical Sciences

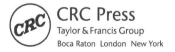

CRC Press
Taylor & Francis Group
Boca Raton London New York

CRC Press is an imprint of the
Taylor & Francis Group, an **informa** business

CRC Press
Taylor & Francis Group
6000 Broken Sound Parkway NW, Suite 300
Boca Raton, FL 33487-2742

© 2000 by Taylor & Francis Group, LLC
CRC Press is an imprint of Taylor & Francis Group, an Informa business

No claim to original U.S. Government works

Visit the Taylor & Francis Web site at
http://www.taylorandfrancis.com

and the CRC Press Web site at
http://www.crcpress.com

Printed and bound by CPI Group (UK) Ltd, Croydon, CR0 4YY

Preface

We have designed this book as a review both for students currently enrolled in a microbiology course and for students who are reviewing microbiology in preparation for the USMLE Part 1. We think the questions cover the most important areas of the various subdisciplines of microbiology. The percentage of questions in immunology, virology, bacteriology, pathogenic bacteria, mycology and parasitology are roughly comparable to the distribution of questions in recent USMLE Part 1 examinations.

The book is laid out so that you can cover the answers as you read and try to answer each question. After making your choice, we suggest you uncover the answer only. If your choice was wrong, try to figure out why before looking at the explanation. Even after you have chosen the correct answer, it is important to read the annotation to the answer because it will briefly describe the key points underlying the question.

Newly emerging infections, development of antibiotic resistance by old adversaries, advances in molecular biology, and new treatments based on stimulation of the immune system, all converge to make microbiology one of the most important disciplines in preparing for a medical career during the first half of the new millennium. We hope this review helps consolidate your knowledge in this area.

Good luck.

Contents

Contents

Number in parentheses indicates number of questions available.

Acknowledgements

The students in Medical Microbiology at the Medical College of Georgia, who first saw these questions as part of their examinations. Their feedback and comments refined and clarified the original questions to produce those you see here.

The faculty of the Department of Immunology and Microbiology at the Medical College of Georgia whose help and support made us all better teachers. Special thanks to Catherine Roesel (PhD), unfortunately now retired, who served as a role model of a committed, superb teacher. Thanks also to David Lapp (PhD) for reviewing the parasitology section.

Dr Thomas R. Gest, Series Editor and former colleague who trusted us to prepare a review book consistent with the high standards of the series.

Andy C. Reese, PhD
Cherukantath N. Nair, PhD
George H. Brownell, PhD

I.   GENERAL IMMUNOLOGY

Non-specific Host Defenses

For questions 1–5, choose the single best answer.

1. Which of the following is characteristic of acute inflammation?
    A. Accumulation of PMNs
    B. Accumulation of mast cells
    C. Accumulation of macrophages
    D. Decreased blood flow due to capillary collapse
    E. Endothelial cell proliferation

A is correct.
PMNs are attracted by various chemotactic factors. Mast cells and macrophages are rare in inflammatory sites. Blood flow *increases*, which produces the red color and heat of an inflamed area.

2. Which of the following is NOT characteristic of eosinophils?
    A. The major component of their specific granules is major basic protein
    B. They have few lysosomes
    C. They are about 8–10 µm in diameter with very little cytoplasm
    D. Their most important function is to kill intracellular bacteria such as *Mycobacterium*
    E. One of their most important killing mechanisms involves NO

D is correct.
Major basic protein, the most important factor in killing parasites, makes up about 50% of the protein in the specific granules. The few lysosomes that are present supplement the activity of major basic protein.

3. Which of the following occurs first during an inflammatory response?
    A. Arrival of neutrophils at the site
    B. Vasodilation of capillaries
    C. Release of migration inhibition factor
    D. Stimulation of mast cell degranulation
    E. Induction of adhesion molecule expression on endothelial cells

E is correct.
While it is true that inflammation releases chemotactic factors for PMNs, they must adhere to adhesion molecules on the endothelial cells before they can move out of the capillaries to the site of inflammation. Indeed, inflammation also stimulates the PMNs to express the reciprocal adhesion molecules needed to bind to the adhesion molecules on the endothelial cells.

4. Which of the following cells is most important in initiating an inflammatory reaction?
    A. Monocytes
    B. Neutrophils
    C. Mast cells
    D. Endothelial cells
    E. Eosinophils

C is correct.
Mast cells are the only ones listed that release large amounts of vasoactive amines and factors chemotactic for eosinophils and neutrophils.

5. Which of the following is NOT a mechanism by which commensal bacteria prevent growth of pathogenic bacteria?
    A. They use up the available oxygen
    B. They produce antimicrobial factors
    C. They occupy all available ecological niches
    D. They use up available nutrients
    E. They secrete bases which make the environment too alkaline for most pathogens

E is correct.
Commensal bacteria are more likely to secrete acids than bases. The importance of commensal bacteria in protecting against pathogens is seen in the not infrequent infections with low grade pathogens following antibiotic treatment that kills the commensal bacteria.

Complement

For questions 6–11, choose the single best answer.

6. CR3 receptors bind to bacteria coated with:
    A. C3a
    B. C3b
    C. iC3b
    D. C3d
    E. C5b

C is correct.
CR1 binds to C3b and CR2 binds to C3d. The others are not recognized by CR receptors.

7. Which of the following is chemotactic for polymorphonuclear neutrophils (PMNs)?
    A. C5a
    B. C3b
    C. IL-12
    D. IFN-γ
    E. IgG

A is correct.
C5a is one of the most potent chemotactic factors known. C3b and IgG are opsonins with no chemotactic activity. IL-12 has no chemotactic activity; however, IL-8 (produced by stimulated macrophage-lineage cells and endothelial cells) is strongly chemotactic for PMNs. IFN-γ activates PMNs but does not induce directional migration.

8. Properdin is important in which of the following?
    A. Inhibiting the activity of C1s esterase
    B. Stabilizing the C3bBb complex
    C. Initiating the alternative (properdin) pathway
    D. Splitting C3a and C5a to inactivate them
    E. Opsonizing bacteria for removal by macrophages

B is correct.
The C3bBb complex is unstable, so it falls apart within a few seconds. Stabilization with properdin allows it to remain together and functional for several minutes. C1 esterase inhibitor (INH) is the factor that inhibits C1s. The alternative pathway is initiated by BC3b binding to endotoxin on the gram-negative bacteria.

9. Patients deficient in C8 have an increased incidence of which of the following?
    A. Infections with *E. coli*
    B. Mucocutaneous candidiasis
    C. Meningitis due to *Neisseria*
    D. Chronic granulomatous disease (CGD)
    E. Chronic inflammatory reactions due to the build up of anaphylatoxins

C is correct.
The lytic part of the pathway seems to be particularly important for protection against gram-negative bacteria of the genus *Neisseria*. *E. coli* is a gram-negative bacterium, but it is normally handled relatively well by neutrophils.

10. Carboxypeptidase N inactivates which of the following?
    A. C1q
    B. Properdin
    C. C3b
    D. C5a
    E. The membrane attack complex

D is correct.
It inactivates both C3a and C5a by splitting the C-terminal arginine from each molecule.

11. Which part of the membrane attack complex actually polymerizes in the membrane to form a transmembrane channel?
    A. C5b
    B. C6
    C. C7
    D. C8
    E. C9

E is correct.
All of the components listed are part of the complex, but only C9 has a tail that penetrates through the cell membrane. It polymerizes in a circle to leave a channel through the middle. Binding of C8 may make the membrane 'leaky' but no channel is formed.

Antigen Binding Molecules

For questions 12–16, match the lettered immunoglobulin class with the appropriate numbered statement.
    A. IgM
    B. IgG
    C. IgA
    D. IgE
    E. IgD

12. The first immunoglobulin synthesized in response to an initial exposure to an antigen in food.

A is correct.
We tend to think (correctly) of IgA being produced in the gut-associated mucosal tissues. However, IgM is produced first in the mucosal-associated tissues as in the other lymphoid tissues, but in the gut-associated lymphoid tissues the switch is preferentially to IgA rather than IgG.

13. The immunoglobulin that has four subclasses.

B is correct.
IgG is not only the immunoglobulin present in highest concentration in circulation, but it also has the most subclasses. IgA and IgE have two subclasses each.

14. Most important in protecting a 2-month-old baby from common bacteria.

B is correct.
It is true that the baby is *making* mostly IgM at that age. However, most of its protection is from IgG transferred across the placenta prior to birth.

15. Of particular importance in protecting against an infestation with schistosomes.

D is correct.
The inflammatory response appears to be particularly important in protecting against helminthes infestations. IgE is the only class that can directly stimulate the inflammatory response.

16. The major immunoglobulin in immune globulin.

B is correct.
The circulating half-life of the other immunoglobulins is too short to be useful in treating immune deficiencies.

For questions 17–19, choose the single best answer.

17.   MHC class III genes code for all the following EXCEPT:
   A. TNFα
   B. C4
   C. Complement component B
   D. Properdin
   E. C2

D is correct.
Note that the complement components coded in this region are those that form the C3 convertases (C4 and C2 form classical C3 convertase, whereas B is part of the alternate pathway C3 convertase).

18.   The affinity of an antibody is a measure of:
   A. How well it is bound by Fc receptors on phagocytes and mast cells
   B. The strength of its binding to an antigen
   C. How far it moves during electrophoresis
   D. The number of antigens it can bind
   E. Its ability to neutralize toxins

B is correct.
Avidity depends on a combination of affinity and the number of antigen binding sites, i.e. ten for IgM, four for IgA, and two for IgG.

19.   Which of the following is NOT a mechanism by which IgA protects us?
   A. Activation of complement via the alternative pathway to lyse gram-negative bacteria
   B. Agglutination of bacteria to make it more difficult for them to penetrate the mucosal surface
   C. Binding with the active site of toxins to inactivate them
   D. Opsonizing bacteria for recognition and phagocytosis by PMNs
   E. Neutralizing viruses by binding to their attachment molecules

D is correct.
Phagocytes have receptors only for IgG, so it is the only class that can induce antibody-dependent cellular cytotoxicity.

For questions 20–23, match the statement with the appropriate lettered fragment or enzyme from the figure below.

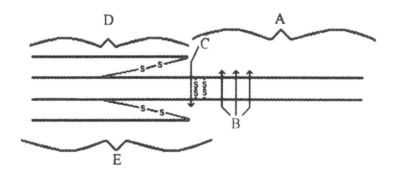

20.   The point(s) at which pepsin splits the molecule.

B is correct.
Pepsin splits the second constant domain into several fragments.

21.   Fc portion.

A is correct.
Fc stands for fragment crystalizable. It is this portion of the IgG molecule that is recognized and bound by receptors on phagocytes.

22. Fab.

D is correct.
The action of papain splits the molecule at C producing two fragments that retain the ability to bind antigen (fragment antigen binding) and the Fc piece.

23. F(ab')₂

E is correct.
Pepsin splits the heavy chains on the COOH terminal side of the intrachain disulfide bonds, so it leaves the two antigen binding pieces linked together. They also have a few extra amino acids.

For questions 24–27, choose the single best answer.

24. Which of the following is NOT true of IgG?
    A. Fixes complement
    B. Crosses the placenta to provide protection to the newborn baby
    C. Opsonizes targets for removal by phagocytes
    D. Neutralizes viruses
    E. Is actively transported into external secretions such as saliva

E is correct.
Some or all of the IgG subclasses are involved in all of the other activities. IgG is found in external secretions, but it is passively transferred, not actively transported as is IgA.

25. How many germline genes are transcribed to form a complete IgG molecule?
    A. 4
    B. 5
    C. 6
    D. 7
    E. 8

D is correct.
Heavy chains require V, D, J and C genes. Light chains require separate V, J and C genes.

26. Allergen-specific IgE is normally measured with:
    A. Latex bead agglutination
    B. Complement fixation test
    C. Countercurrent electrophoresis
    D. Coombs' test
    E. RAST

E is correct.
RAST stands for the radioallergosorbant test. It uses radiolabeled anti-IgE antibodies to quantify the amount of serum IgE bound to an immobilized allergen. The other tests listed are not sensitive enough to measure the picogram levels of allergen-specific IgE even if the test could be adapted for the purpose.

27. Electrostatic interactions between antigen and antibody implies that a positive charge on the antigen epitope will be matched by:
    A. A positive charge in the paratope of the antibody
    B. A negative charge in the paratope of the antibody
    C. No charge in the paratope of the antibody
    D. A depression in the paratope of the antibody into which the positive charge can fit
    E. A hydrophobic region in the paratope of the antibody

B is correct.
Like charges repel and unlike charges attract. A hydrophobic region is essentially the same as an electrically neutral region. A depression in the paratope would match a protrusion in the antigenic determinant.

Lymphocytes and Lymphoid Tissues

For questions 28–30, match the lettered cell type with the appropriate numbered statement.

  A. T cells
  B. B cells
  C. NK cells
  D. Both T and B cells
  E. All of the above

28. CD3 is a marker found on which of the cells?

A is correct.
CD3 is the part of the T-cell receptor complex that signals to the inside of the cell that an antigen is bound to the T-cell receptor itself. Carrying the signal across the cell membrane is called *transduction*.

29. The cells which have class I HLA (MHC) antigens on their cytoplasmic membranes.

E is correct.
HLA class I molecules are the 'self' markers. They are found on all nucleated cells. They express antigens that are synthesized within the cell. Since viral infections and cancers trigger the cell to make antigens not normally found on the affected cell, HLA class I molecules are key parts of the immune system response to viral infections and cancers.

30. Which cell type(s) express antigen-specific receptors?

D is correct.
Part of the definition of a mature T or B cell is the expression of antigen-specific receptors. NK cells are part of the body's non-specific defense system since they lack antigen receptors.

For questions 31–47, choose the single best answer.

31. MHC class II proteins are normally found on which of the following cells?
  A. All cells
  B. All nucleated cells
  C. Antigen presenting cells (including B cells)
  D. Endothelial cells
  E. Phagocytic cells

C is correct.
The major function of class II molecules is to present exogenous antigen to helper T cells.

32. What percentage of peripheral T cells has the γδ receptor?
  A. 0
  B. <2%
  C. 5–15%
  D. ~50%
  E. >90%

C is correct.
However, the function of γδT cells is largely unknown.

33. Transduction of the signal that the TCR has bound an antigen is via which component?
    A. TCRα chain
    B. TCRβ chain
    C. CD3
    D. CD4
    E. CD8

C is correct.
The part of CD3 that actually carries the signal is the η–ζ or ζ–ζ dimer. The cytoplasmic tails of the α and β chains are not long enough to carry the signal. CD4 and CD8 are the receptors for MHC class II and class I proteins, respectively.

34. Which of the following is considered a primary lymphoid organ?
    A. Thymus
    B. Lymph node
    C. Spleen
    D. Tonsil
    E. Liver

A is correct.
Primary lymphoid organs are those in which lymphocytes mature to functional effector cells. T cells mature in the thymus under the influence of several thymic hormones of which thymosin, thymopoietin and thymulin are the best known. Bone marrow (in humans) or the bursa of Fabricius (in birds) are the sites of B-cell maturation.

35. Which of the following could be used to identify B cells in a mixture of lymphocytes?
    A. Lymphoproliferative response to concanavalin A
    B. Determination of surface Fc receptors
    C. Lymphoproliferative response to phytohemagglutin
    D. Determination of surface CD2 via erythrocyte rosettes
    E. Determination of C' receptors

E is correct.
Both B cells and T cells have Fc receptors. Answers A, C and D are specific for T cells.

36. Which cells are responsible for most instances of antibody-dependent cellular cytotoxicity (ADCC)?
    A. T cells
    B. K cells
    C. Eosinophils
    D. NK cells
    E. Plasma cells

B is correct.
ADCC requires receptors on the effector cell for IgG, and the ability of the effector cell to secrete lytic factors. Killer (K) cells are the only ones in this group that fit that description.

37. Which of the following are not MHC-restricted in the mechanism by which they kill non-opsonized, virally infected cells?
    A. Monocytes
    B. Cytotoxic T cells
    C. Interferons
    D. NK cells
    E. Neutrophils

D is correct.
T cells kill virally infected cells but are MHC-restricted, i.e. they recognize viral antigens presented by MHC proteins. Monocytes and neutrophils are not able to recognize virally infected cells unless they are coated with antibody. IFNs inhibit viral replication, but do not kill the infected cells.

38. Long-term transfer of immunity can be achieved by transferring which of the following from an immunized animal to a naive animal?
    A. Phagocytes
    B. Lymphocytes
    C. Antibodies
    D. Cytokines
    E. Acute phase reactants

B is correct.
Antibodies confer short-term protection, but only lymphocytes provide the long-term protection.

39. Most of the antibody in circulation comes from:
    A. T cells
    B. B cells
    C. Plasma cells
    D. NK cells
    E. All of the above

C is correct.
Only B cells and plasma cells make antibody, but plasma cells make by far the greatest amount.

40. B cells are found in higher concentrations than T cells in which tissues?
    A. Cortex of lymph nodes
    B. Blood
    C. Periarterial cuff of the spleen
    D. The halo around germinal centers in tonsils
    E. Lymph

A is correct.
B cells are found in each of the other tissues, but they are greatly outnumbered by T cells.

41. Which of the following cells proliferate in the presence of liposaccharide (LPS)?
    A. T cells
    B. B cells
    C. NK cells
    D. Both T and B cells
    E. All of the above

B is correct.
LPS interacts with receptors on mouse B cells and directly with the membrane to send both signals necessary to activate B cells. T cells and NK cells lack the LPS receptors, so they are not affected.

42. Which of the following cell types directly initiates the phospholipase C–IP$_3$ pathway following allosteric change induced by antigen binding to the antigen receptor?
    A. T-cell receptor (α and β chains)
    B. CD3
    C. CD4
    D. CD8
    E. IL-2 receptor

B is correct.
The cytoplasmic tails of CD3 have sequences with phosphatase activity that activate tyrosine kinases which, in turn, activate phospholipase C.

43. The portion of the T-cell receptor complex that provides the 'second signal' in cytotoxic T cells is:
    A. CD2
    B. CD3
    C. β chain of the receptor
    D. CD8
    E. LFA-1

D is correct.
CD8 is a member of the immunoglobulin superfamily and is found only on Tc cells. Binding to the MHC class I molecule causes activation of a protein kinase on the cytoplasmic tail of the CD8 molecule.

44. The first component of the immune system to appear during fetal development is:
    A. IgM
    B. T cells
    C. Complement
    D. B cells
    E. NK cells

B is correct.
T cells develop slightly earlier than B cells during immune development. Of course B cells are necessary to produce immunoglobulins such as IgM. Complement and NK cells are not part of the immune system proper, although they may be activated by immune products.

45. All of the following are members of the immunoglobulin superfamily EXCEPT:
    A. TCRβ chain
    B. β2-microglobulin
    C. CD4
    D. CR1 (complement receptor 1)
    E. MHC class II

D is correct.
It is true that members of the immunoglobulin superfamily are mostly involved in recognition reactions. However, CR1 does not share the typical disulfide stabilized domain structure of the family. β2-microglobulin is essentially a single domain that some have hypothesized is the original member of the family. Other members include CD8 and Thy1.

46. Which of the following is the component on the T cell that actually binds to the antigen?
    A. T-cell receptor (α and β chains)
    B. CD3
    C. CD4
    D. CD8
    E. IL-2 receptor

A is correct.
Both the α and β chains have variable regions arising from gene rearrangement similar to that of B cells. These variable regions interact to form the specific antigen binding site.

47. The receptor for CD2 is:
    A. Sialyl Lewis^x
    B. ICAM-1
    C. VLA-5
    D. LFA-3
    E. CD28

D is correct.
Each of these molecules is important in cell–cell interactions in host defenses. Sialyl Lewis^x binds to P-selectin; ICAM-1 binds to LFA-1; VLA-5 binds to fibronectin; CD28 binds to B7 (CD80). LFA-1, VLA-5 and fibronectin are members of the integrin superfamily. CD2, CD28 and LFA-1 are all on T cells and are important in providing additional activation signals to supplement the signal sent by antigen binding.

Lymphocyte Maturation

For questions 48–51, choose the single best answer.

48. In humans, B-cell maturation occurs in the:
    A. Bursa of Fabricius
    B. Bone marrow
    C. Blood circulation
    D. B-cell areas of the gut-associated lymphoid tissues
    E. They are mature when they are formed from the lymphocyte stem cell

B is correct.
Humans do not have a bursa of Fabricius although it is the site of B-cell maturation in birds. In humans, B cells leave the bone marrow as mature, antigen reactive cells.

49. Which of the following occurs earliest in maturation of T cells in the thymus?
    A. Expression of CD3
    B. Rearrangement of TCR α chain
    C. Rearrangement of TCR β chain
    D. Expression of CD4
    E. Expression of CD8

C is correct.
This event triggers expression of CD4 *and* CD8 followed by α chain rearrangement and finally CD3 expression.

50. In the thymus, lymphocytes are induced to undergo apoptosis under what conditions?
    A. They encounter class I MHC (HLA) antigens on dendritic cells
    B. They encounter class II MHC (HLA) antigens on macrophages
    C. They encounter an antigen–MHC complex to which they can bind strongly
    D. They rearrange the α chain of the T-cell receptor
    E. They encounter thymosin

C is correct.
This is the major way the body prevents development of T cells that can react to self antigens because the antigens encountered in the thymus are overwhelmingly self antigens. Interaction with class I and II MHC antigens is necessary for T-cell development.

51. Proliferation of lymphocytes in the thymus:
    A. Produces many more lymphocytes than ever leave the thymus
    B. Is antigen driven
    C. Stops after rearrangement of the genes to form a functional T-cell antigen receptor
    D. Has a generation time of 48–72 hours
    E. Applies only to lymphocytes that have αβ receptors but not those with γδ receptors

A is correct.
Most of the lymphocytes generated in the thymus die there, at least part of which is due to deletion of self-reactive cells. The proliferation rate is hormonally induced and very rapid, with a division time of about 12 hours. Proliferation continues until the T cells are mature and ready to exit the thymus.

Antigens and Tests for Antigens and Antibodies

For questions 52–59, choose the single best answer.

52. A hapten:
    A. Stimulates T-cell responses
    B. Stimulates B-cell responses
    C. Enhances the response of an antigen by forming a depot for the antigen
    D. Activates macrophages for increased phagocytosis
    E. Requires a carrier to initiate an immune response

E is correct.
A hapten is too small to be processed and expressed on the antigen-presenting cell. When it is coupled to a larger molecule, the whole complex is processed and expressed. The free hapten can then be recognized by the appropriate antigen receptors.

53. Adjuvants may be used to:
    A. Form a depot for the antigen, thereby enhancing the immune response to the antigen
    B. Suppress the immune response to self antigens
    C. Inhibit the inflammatory response
    D. Attract PMNs and macrophages to the site of an infection
    E. Stimulate Tc cell responses to viruses

A is correct.
This is the most common mechanism of action of adjuvants. The slow, continuous release of the antigen from the depot provides more opportunity for the appropriate antigen-presenting cells and lymphocytes to encounter and respond to the antigen.

54. What information can NOT be obtained from analysis with a cytofluorograph?
    A. The size of the cell
    B. Which stage of the cell proliferation cycle the cell is in
    C. Whether there were immune complexes deposited in a tissue slide of the kidney
    D. Whether particular cell surface antigens were present on the cell
    E. The number of CD4$^+$ and CD8$^+$ cells present in the blood of a suspected AIDS patient

C is correct.
The cytofluorograph measures characteristics of cells in suspension.

55. Which of the following tests is the LEAST sensitive?
    A. Agglutination
    B. Nephelometry
    C. Flow cytometry
    D. Radial immunodiffusion
    E. Countercurrent electrophoresis

D is correct.
Tests that depend on lattice formation of soluble antigens are the least sensitive tests. Countercurrent electrophoresis is more sensitive than RID because it focuses the antigen available, whereas the antigen concentration in RID decreases with the square of the radius of the circle.

56. Which of the following antigen–antibody pairs would produce a visible precipitate in the bottom of a test tube?
    A. Monoclonal antibody to human albumin and human serum
    B. Antiserum to metabolites of cocaine and urine from an athlete who was a regular user of crack
    C. Antiserum to pentadecylcatechol (the allergen in poison ivy) and a concentrated extract of poison ivy leaves
    D. Rabbit anti-human IgG3 and serum from a healthy 81-year-old woman

D is correct.
A visible precipitate requires lattice formation. Monoclonal antibody does not produce a lattice because it can bind to only one determinant on an antigen. Quantities of cocaine metabolites in urine are too low to form a lattice. Pentadecyl-catechol is a hapten, i.e. it has only one determinant so it cannot be crosslinked. A healthy 81-year-old would have abundant levels of IgG3.

57. The Ouchterlony (double diffusion in agar) test would be the test of choice for which of the following?
    A. Measure the concentration of cocaine metabolites in urine of an athlete
    B. Screen serum for myeloma immunoglobulin(s)
    C. Determine the D (Rh$^+$) antigen on erythrocytes
    D. Distinguish human from chicken blood at a crime scene
    E. Measure serum IgE

D is correct.
The pattern at the intersection of precipitin lines produced by anti-human hemoglobin to the unknown and known human hemoglobin would allow one to make the distinction. The Ouchterlony test is not sensitive enough to measure drug metabolites or IgE. Serum components are compared using immuno-electrophoresis.

58. A paratope:
    A. Is the part of the antibody that binds to the antigenic determinant
    B. Is the part of the antigen that makes actual contact with the antibody
    C. Is usually an alpha helix
    D. Defines the subclass of IgG immunoglobulins
    E. Is the part of the antigen that is bound by the MHC class II molecule

A is correct.
The antigen binding site on an antibody consists of amino acids in the hypervariable regions of heavy and light chains which does not include an alpha helix.

59. Which of the following is true of the enzyme linked immunosorbant assay?
    A. It is commonly used to screen for an abnormal protein(s) in a complex mixture such as serum
    B. It is the assay of choice for measuring growth hormone in an undersized child
    C. It can be used to trace a nerve tract through a muscle
    D. It is read in a microscope equipped with a UV light source
    E. It depends on lattice formation with the antigen and antibody

B is correct.
It is very sensitive so it is a good choice for measuring substances in low concentration such as growth hormone. Its sensitivity is precisely because it does not depend on lattice formation. It is measured in a special spectrophotometer, so it cannot be easily used to measure tissue antigens.

For questions 60 and 61, base your answers on the following figure:

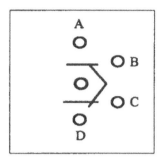

60.   If the above Ouchterlony pattern was generated using antiserum to adult hemoglobin in the center well, which pair of wells could contain fetal hemoglobin and adult hemoglobin, respectively?
   A. A and B
   B. B and C
   C. C and D

A is correct.
This is the classic partial identity pattern. The antiserum would recognize the α chain present in both types of hemoglobin. However, it would recognize the β chain of adult hemoglobin (in well A) that is not present in fetal hemoglobin (well B). Note the spur points to the well deficient in determinants recognized by the antiserum.

61.   If the above Ouchterlony pattern was generated using antisera to hemoglobin isolated from cord blood, which pair of wells could contain fetal hemoglobin and adult hemoglobin, respectively?
   A. A and B
   B. B and C
   C. C and D

C is correct.
Cord blood contains both fetal and adult hemoglobin, so antibodies would be made against the α, β and γ chains. Antibodies to the β chain of the adult would not be precipitated by the fetal hemoglobin. Similarly, antibodies to the γ chain of the fetal hemoglobin would not be precipitated by the adult hemoglobin. The result is the formation of two spurs which look like lines of non-identity even though the two types of hemoglobin share a common α chain.

Cellular Control of Immune Responses

For questions 62–69, choose the single best answer.

62.   Which class of immunoglobulin would be induced by injection of inactivated cholera toxin in a T cell-deficient mouse?
   A. IgM
   B. IgG
   C. IgA
   D. IgE
   E. IgD

A is correct.
Not much immunoglobulin of any kind would be made, but IgM is less T cell-dependent than other classes.

63.   Which of the following stabilizes contact with cells bearing MHC class II?
   A. T-cell receptor (α and β chains)
   B. CD3
   C. CD4
   D. CD8
   E. IL-1 receptor

C is correct.
CD8 binds to MHC class I molecules. CD3 transduces a signal that the TCR has bound antigen.

64. Which of the following carry endogenous peptides from the cytoplasm to the endoplasmic reticulum lumen where they associate with MHC class I proteins?
    A. Invariant chain
    B. MHC class II proteins
    C. β2-microglobulin
    D. C5a
    E. TAP1 and TAP2

E is correct.
TAP stands for transporter of antigenic peptides. Invariant chain binds to the antigen binding grove in MHC class II proteins until they fuse with a phagolysosome where enzymes digest the invariant chain. This frees the class II protein to bind to an antigen fragment in the phago-lysosome.

65. Th1 cells inhibit development of Th2 cells by secreting which of the following cytokines?
    A. IL-2
    B. IL-4
    C. IL-6
    D. TNF-β
    E. IFN-γ

E is correct.
Th0 cells can differentiate into either Th1 or Th2 cells. IFN-γ is made by Th1 cells and prevents Th2 development, thereby maintaining the delayed hypersensitivity-type responses induced by Th1 cells.

66. Which of the following is true of T suppressor cells?
    A. They probably represent reciprocal inhibition by Th1 and Th2 cells
    B. They inhibit PMNs and macrophages
    C. They are always CD8+
    D. They secrete antigen-specific suppressor factors
    E. T cells with suppressor function do not exist

A is correct.
Th1 cells secrete IFNγ which inhibits development of Th2 cells. TH2 cells produce IL-10 which inhibits Th1 development. Many of the experiments that pointed to the existence of suppressor cells did not take this type of reciprocal inhibition into account because it was unknown at the time. Thus suppressor cells exist, but probably not cells that have suppression as their only function.

67. Clonal selection implies:
    A. The pre-existence of lymphocytes with receptors specific for the antigen
    B. That clones of bacteria are eliminated more quickly than heterogeneous infections
    C. That monoclonal antibodies could be produced to treat cancers since they usually are a clone of a single transformed cell
    D. That antigens serve as a template which instructs lymphocytes to produce complementary antibodies (a clone of antibodies)
    E. None of the above

A is correct.
Lymphoid tissues are distributed such that they maximize contact between antigens and lymphocytes. The antigen finally encounters a lymphocyte with receptors that are specific for it. The receptors arise from almost random rearrangement of germ line genes, so there is no place in the process for the antigen to induce receptors specific for itself.

68. Which of the following cells is considered the most important in antigen processing and presentation?
    A. Neutrophils
    B. Langerhans cells
    C. Endothelial cells
    D. T cells
    E. Thymic epithelial cells

B is correct.
The monocyte–macrophage lineage cells are considered the pre-eminent antigen presenting cells.

69. Which of the following do NOT require antigen processing and presentation by APCs?
    A. Tc cells
    B. Th1 cells
    C. Th2 cells
    D. B cells

A is correct.
Tc cells respond to antigen in association with MHC class I proteins so APC processing and expression are not necessary. The other cells must see antigen in association with MHC class II molecules.

Cytokines and Hormones

For questions 70–75, match the lettered cytokine with the appropriate numbered statement.

A. IL-1
B. IL-2
C. IL-6
D. IL-10
E. IFN-γ

70. Inhibits Th1 cells.

D is correct.
IL-10 is produced primarily by Th2 cells and inhibits the activity of Th1 cells. Conversely, IFN-γ is made mostly by Th1 cells and inhibits Th2 cell activity.

71. Required for B-cell maturation to plasma cells.

C is correct.
Several of the cytokines, e.g. IL-4 and IL-5, are growth factors for B cells, but IL-6 seems to be particularly important in the differentiation of B cells to plasma cells.

72. The primary growth factor for T cells.

B is correct.
The original name for IL-2 was T-cell growth factor. It is a powerful growth factor for all types of T cells.

73. The most potent macrophage activator.

E is correct.
IL-2 does have some activity as a macrophage activator, but it is not nearly as potent as IFN-γ. The other cytokines have no macrophage-activating activity.

74. Stimulates synthesis and release of acute-phase proteins.

C is correct.
Acute phase proteins are a group of protective serum proteins whose concentration is increased by 10- to 1000-fold during an inflammatory response. This is an important way in which immune responses make use of pre-existing non-specific defenses to provide protection for the host.

75. Provides the 'second signal' to stimulate Th cells to become activated and proliferate.

A is correct.
The first signal is provided by cross-linking of the Th cell antigen receptor. If the Th cell does not receive a second activating signal shortly after the first signal, it undergoes apoptosis. Activating other receptors, e.g. CD4 or B7, can also provide the second signal.

For questions 76–81, choose the single best answer.

76.   One probable mechanism for the placebo effect is that our belief in the efficacy of a drug:
  A. Stimulates Ts cells
  B. Induces production of IL-2 and IL-6
  C. Alters the pattern of neuropeptide secretion such that normal immune responses are restored
  D. Activates professional phagocytes (PMNs and macrophages) to greater activity
  E. Makes us *feel* better but has no effect on the underlying problem

C is correct.
Neuropeptides control much of the immune response just as they do most other body responses. Our beliefs and perceptions influence the production of various neurohormones.

77.   Which of the neurohormones inhibits Th1 cells but not Th2 cells?
  A. Vasoactive intestinal peptide (VIP)
  B. Growth hormone
  C. Adrenocorticotropic hormone (ACTH)
  D. Substance P
  E. Thyroid stimulating hormone (TSH)

C is correct.
VIP has just the opposite effect. Growth hormone, substance P and TSH are stimulatory for all cellular responses. Of course, ACTH also stimulates cortisone which suppresses lymphocyte formation.

78.   Which of the following acts by inducing apoptosis in its target cells?
  A. IL-4
  B. IFN-γ
  C. Perforin
  D. Transfer factor
  E. TNF-β

E is correct.
Perforin acts similarly to C9 of complement in that it makes holes in the target-cell membrane. The other cytokines are not directly cytotoxic.

79.   Which of the following factors secreted by macrophages induces the target cell to undergo apoptosis?
  A. IL-1
  B. TNF-α
  C. IFN-α
  D. H_2O_2
  E. Lysozyme

B is correct.
TNF-α and its first cousin, TNF-β, initiate the process of apoptosis in the target cells. The other factors listed may have direct toxic effects on the target (H_2O_2 and lysozyme) or activate other systems to greater protective activity (IL-1 and INF-α).

80.   Which of the following cytokines stimulates a class switch to IgE?
  A. IL-2
  B. IL-4
  C. IL-5
  D. IL-6
  E. IFN-γ

B is correct.
IL-4 alone seems to stimulate IgE synthesis, whereas the other classes seem to require multiple cytokines. For example IL-4, IL-5 and IL-6 together stimulate IgG synthesis.

81.   Stress effects on the immune system are mediated mostly by:
  A. Substance P
  B. Cortisol
  C. Leuteinizing hormone (LH)
  D. Growth hormone
  E. Androsterone

B is correct.
Cortisol generally suppresses lymphocyte development and function. ACTH which induces the cortisone synthesis and secretion is also suppressive.

For questions 82–85, match the statement with the appropriate lettered cytokine.

   A. IL-1
   B. IL-4
   C. IL-6
   D. IL-10
   E. IFN-γ

82.   Most potent stimulator of MHC class II expression on B cells and macrophages.

E is correct.
Both IL-4 and IFN-γ induce MHC class II expression, but IFN-γ is much stronger.

83.   Directs the immune response toward humoral and delayed hypersensitivity responses by inhibiting the activity and/or development of Th2 cells.

E is correct.
IL-10 and IFN-γ form a mutual inhibitory loop. IL-10 inhibits Th1 cells which synthesize IFN-γ. On the other hand, IFN-γ inhibits Th2 cells that synthesize IL-10.

84.   Stimulates production of stem cells that are the precursors for all types of leukocytes.

C is correct.
Most of the interleukins have growth-stimulating effects for one or more cell types. IL-6 acts on, among others, hemopoietic stem cells.

85.   Provides the second signal to Th cells after they have bound antigen.

A is correct.
IL-1 is highly pleiotropic with many functions in both the immune response and other systems. In the immune response, it provides the second signal without which Th cells will undergo apoptosis.

II.   CLINICAL IMMUNOLOGY

Effector Functions of the Immune System

For questions 86–94, choose the single best answer.

86.   Which of the following is true for the T-cell secondary response?
   A. It produces much greater levels of cytokines than the primary response
   B. It takes about 5–7 days to be manifest because the cells have to proliferate and then make and secrete the cytokines
   C. It is operative only with delayed hypersensitivity responses (Th1 cells)
   D. It shuts down more quickly than the primary response because it is more effective at eliminating the pathogen than the primary response
   E. It does not require antigen to be presented in association with an MHC protein

A is correct.
General characteristics of both T- and B-cell secondary responses are that they are induced by lower levels of antigen than the primary response, produce more effector substances (cytokines or antibody) more quickly, and last longer. All types of T cells produce memory cells, the basis of secondary responses, but memory cells still need to see the MHC–Ag complex.

87.   Which of the following factors is NOT secreted by macrophages?
   A. IFN-α
   B. TNF-α
   C. IL-1
   D. Prostaglandin E_1
   E. IL-2

E is correct.
The most important source of IL-2 in the immune response is Th1 cells, although many other cells can make it. TNF-α is a major cytotoxic factor secreted by macrophages. Virally infected leukocytes produce IFN-α. IL-1 is the most pleiotropic of the interleukins. Its major function in the immune response is to provide the second signal to activate T cells. Prostaglandin E_1 generally suppresses cell growth, so it is one of the mechanisms by which macrophages inhibit cancer growth.

88.   Chronic mucocutaneous candidiasis (fungal infection) would result from:
   A. Inadequate circulating B cells
   B. Defective neutrophils
   C. Macrophages that were unable to produce TNF-α and perforin
   D. Non-functional or deficient numbers of Tc cells
   E. Defective Th1 cells or inadequate numbers of Th1 cells

E is correct.
Th1 cells seem to be the most important host defense against fungal infections.

89.   The lag period between primary antigen challenge and appearance of specific antibodies in circulation is approximately:
   A. 6–8 hours
   B. 2–3 days
   C. 5–7 days
   D. 15+ days
   E. Indeterminate; it depends on the nature of the antigen

C is correct.
One might see specific antibodies within a couple of days following a secondary challenge, but a primary challenge produces antibody in a little under a week.

90.   Which of the following is most important in killing of helminths?
   A. Macrophages
   B. Tc cells
   C. Eosinophils
   D. Mast cells
   E. K cells

C is correct.
Major basic proteins from eosinophils seem to be most effective against helminths. However, NO from macrophages is also quite important. Mast cells have little direct effect, but they do help induce an inflammatory response and produce eosinophil chemotactic factor.

91.   Which of the following is the most important mechanism used by trypanosome pathogens to evade host defenses?
   A. Produce prostaglandins that inhibit immune responses
   B. Induce T suppressor cells
   C. Continually change their membrane antigens
   D. Shed large amounts of antigens that overwhelm the immune system
   E. Coat themselves with serum proteins so they look like self

C is correct.
They serially change their major surface antigens, so by the time the immune system has made antibody to one set, it has been replaced by another.

92.   The receptor for HIV is:
   A. CD3
   B. CD4
   C. CD8
   D. Gp120
   E. CR2 (complement receptor 2)

B is correct.
Since CD4 is the marker for T helper cells, HIV wipes out the central cells needed to induce immune responses. CD8 cells are unaffected. Gp120 is the HIV coat protein that binds to the CD4.

93.   Memory cells:
   A. Are always B cells
   B. For IgM and IgG exist in about the same proportions as IgM and IgG in plasma, i.e. about 1:3
   C. Have the same antigen specificity as the originally stimulated B cell
   D. Live only a little longer than naive lymphocytes (lymphocytes that have never been exposed to their antigen)
   E. All of the above

C is correct.
Both T and B memory cells are formed during an immune response. Their ability to prevent reinfection (immunity) depends on the identity of the antigen receptors on descendants of antigen-stimulated lymphocytes. Otherwise, the memory cells would not be able to respond to the pathogen that induced the first illness. The overwhelming majority of B memory cells occur after the immunoglobulin class switch, so few IgM memory cells are formed. One characteristic of memory cells is that they are longer lived than naive cells.

94. Which of the following are most important in killing *M. tuberculosis*?
 A. B cells
 B. T cells
 C. Macrophages
 D. Neutrophils
 E. Membrane attack complex of complement

C is correct.
Intracellular bacteria such as *M. tuberculosis* are somewhat resistant to killing, so macrophages need to be activated by INF-γ from Th1 cells. However, the actual killing is by macrophages. (Neutrophils are not activated by INF-γ and are not very effective in killing intracellular bacteria.)

For question 95, use the following figure of a Western blot.

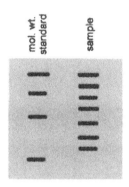

95. The sample is characteristic of a Western blot of DNA from which of the following cells?
 A. Polyploid leukemic cells
 B. Epithelial cells infected with influenza
 C. Cells undergoing apoptosis
 D. Cells infected with an intracellular bacterium such as *Mycobacterium*
 E. Cells killed by complement fixation

C is correct.
Apoptosis induces endonucleases to cut the cell DNA at the nucleosomes, which tends to produce fragments that are multiples of the average nucleosome length. These appear as a 'ladder' on a Western blot.

For questions 96–99, match the statement with the most appropriate cell type.

 A. Th1 cells
 B. Th2 cells
 C. Tc cells
 D. B cells
 E. NK cells

96. Which cells are most important in immunity to measles following immunization with measles virus?

D is correct.
It is true that both B and T memory cells are produced by immunization. However, it is the measles-specific antibody produced by B cells and their descendants the plasma cells that inactivate any new measles viruses before they can infect their target cells. T memory cells do quickly destroy infected cells but usually are not needed.

97.   Which cells are able to immediately react to and destroy many virally infected cells?

E is correct.
NK cells act non-specifically and, therefore, immediately lyse many types of virally infected cells, particularly those of the blood system itself. They do not have specific antigen receptors, so they do not have to proliferate to produce enough cells to be effective against the early stages of a viral infection. If they are completely successful, the person would probably not develop significant symptoms, so he/she would be unaware that a battle was taking place.

98.   Resolution of a herpes lesion on the lip is due to the action of which of the cells?

C is correct.
Herpes is transmitted directly from cell to cell, so it is not exposed to antibody or phagocytic cells. Therefore, it is totally dependent on Tc cells to lyse infected cells and expose the uncoated DNA for destruction by DNAses in the tissue fluids.

99.   Which cells mediate the specific immune response to an initial infection with *Trypanosoma cruzi*?

A is correct.
Th1 cells secrete IFN-γ which stimulates macrophages to kill the parasite. Without this macrophage activating factor, most of the *T. cruzi* are unharmed by the macrophage. Tc cells may lyse infected cells to release the bacteria, so they can be destroyed by the activated macrophages, but that does not seem to be important in host defenses against intracellular pathogens, either bacteria or parasites.

Immune Deficiencies

For questions 100–104, match the statement with the most appropriate defective or absent protein.

   A. Purine nucleoside phosphorylase deficiency
   B. Defective DNA repair mechanisms
   C. Defective or absent CD40
   D. Defective RAG-1 or RAG-2
   E. Defective sialophorin

100.   Wiskott–Aldrich syndrome.

E is correct.
Sialophorin is the ligand for ICAM-1, so its lack inhibits normal regulatory cell interactions.

101.   Hyper-IgM syndrome.

C is correct.
CD40 on the B cell is the ligand for CD40 ligand on activated T cells. The signal generated by CD40 when it is bound is necessary for activation of resting B cells.

102.   Ataxia telangiectasia.

B is correct.
The effects on systems as diverse as the immune system and fine muscle control reflect the ubiquitous importance of DNA repair.

103. Profound T-cell deficiency.

A is correct.
Lack of this enzyme results in an accumulation of dATP and dGTP which are toxic to all cells, but particularly to T cells. Of course, a Th cell deficiency also affects B-cell function, but the primary defect is in T cells.

104. Severe combined immunodeficiency.

D is correct.
These two enzymes (recombination activation gene-products 1 and 2) are needed for the genetic rearrangements that produce immunoglobulins and T-cell antigen receptors. Without them lymphocytes have no antigen receptors.

For questions 105–111, choose the single best answer.

105. A defect in which of the following results in chronic granulomatous disease?
 A. MHC class I proteins
 B. MHC class II proteins
 C. NADPH oxidase of phagocytes
 D. C1 inhibitor
 E. Thymosin

C is correct.
Defects in MHC proteins produce bare leukocyte syndrome. Lack of C1 inhibitor results in angioedema. Thymosin deficiency would result in failure of T-cell maturation.

106. Deficiency of which of the following complement components is most immediately life-threatening?
 A. C1q
 B. C4
 C. Factor B
 D. C5
 E. C7

D is correct.
C3 and C5 are the most important components because both of their split products are biologically active. Deficiencies in C1, C4 and C2 are somewhat ameliorated by the alternative pathway. People with a deficiency in C7 have a higher incidence of meningitis, but it is not as serious as C3 or C5 deficiency.

107. Live virus vaccines cannot be used in which of the following people?
 A. Bruton's agammaglobulinemia
 B. Ataxia telangiectasia
 C. Common variable agammaglobulinemia
 D. Children under 3 years of age
 E. Women with lupus erythematosis

B is correct.
People with T-cell deficiencies have difficulty in clearing viruses, even attenuated ones. The other conditions do not affect T-cell function.

108. The secondary response to *Staphylococcus aureus* is based on:
 A. Formation of memory lymphocytes during the primary response
 B. Enhanced phagocytosis and killing of the *S. aureus* by memory macrophages formed during the primary response
 C. Enhanced phagocytosis and killing of the *S. aureus* by memory PMNs formed during the primary response
 D. Enhanced complement fixation.
 E. All of the above

A is correct.
Only lymphocytes have the ability to 'learn' from previous exposure and become memory cells. More rapid production of IgG antibodies during the secondary response would enhance the phagocytic and complement responses, but the requisite antibody is from memory B cells.

109.   Neutrophils (PMNs) use all of the following to kill phagocytosed bacteria EXCEPT:
   A. Defensins
   B. NO
   C. H_2O_2
   D. Neutral proteases
   E. $O_2^{\bullet}$ (singlet oxygen)

B is correct.
PMNs use all of the other cytotoxic mechanisms including defensins which are small, antimicrobial peptides. NO is an important weapon used by macrophages, but PMNs are unable to generate it.

110.   A severe B-cell deficiency would result in an increased susceptibility to:
   A. AIDS
   B. Chronic mucocutaneous candidiasis
   C. Shingles (herpes zoster infection)
   D. Autoimmune diseases
   E. *Staphylococcus aureus* infections

E is correct.
B-cell deficiency with its resultant immuno-globulin deficiency results in an increased susceptibility to intercellular bacterial infections. *S. aureus* is the only bacterial disease listed.

111.   The first event during germ-line rearrangement for antibody formation is:
   A. Bringing together of the heavy chain D and J genes
   B. Bringing together of the heavy chain V and D genes
   C. Bringing together of the light chain D and J genes
   D. Bringing together of the light chain V and J genes
   E. Bringing together of heavy chain V and J genes

A is correct.
The heavy chain genes rearrange first. If the DJ rearrangement is successful, then the material between the V genes and the DJ genes is removed. When heavy chain rearrangements are successful, the completed heavy chain signals rearrangement of kappa chain genes. If that is unsuccessful, then lambda chain genes are rearranged.

Immunopathology

For questions 112–116, match the statement with the appropriate type of tissue injury.

   A. Type I – allergy
   B. Type II – cytotoxic antibody
   C. Type III – immune complex disease
   D. Type IV – delayed hypersensitivity
   E. Types I, II and III

112.   The type that is absolutely complement dependent.

C is correct.
Type II injury may be exacerbated by complement but is not dependent on it.

113.   Mediated by lymphokines.

D is correct.
Type IV is cell dependent because it requires Th1 cells to produce and release cytokines that attract mononuclear cells to the area and cause them to remain there.

114.   Type of reaction exemplified by the Arthus reaction.

C is correct.
The Arthus reaction results from circulating antibody (from a previous injection) forming immune complexes with intradermal antigen. The C3a and C5a released by complement fixation induce an inflammatory response and subsequent tissue injury.

115.   Type of tissue injury caused by chromium on the posts of ear rings for pierced ears.

D is correct.
Heavy metal reactions are classic delayed hypersensitivity responses.

116.   The type of tissue injury mediated by IgE.

A is correct.
Allergies are mediated by IgE which is bound via the Fc piece to mast cells and basophils. When the surface IgE is cross-linked by allergen, the mast cell or basophil releases its specific granules that contain various vasoactive substances that induce inflammation.

For questions 117–121, choose the single best answer.

117.   Which of the following is the predominant cell type in granulomas?
   A. PMNs
   B. Macrophages
   C. T cells
   D. B cells
   E. Eosinophils

B is correct.
Macrophages are attracted by chemotactic factors released by activated T cells. When they cannot destroy the inducing organism, they continue to accumulate in order to wall it off from the rest of the body.

118.   Asthma is an example of:
   A. An autoimmune disease
   B. Delayed hypersensitivity
   C. An IgE mediated syndrome
   D. An immune complex disease
   E. A combined type II and type III tissue injury

C is correct.
Extrinsic asthma is defined as those asthmatic attacks which are triggered by known allergen(s) and have high IgE levels. However, intrinsic asthma (no known allergen trigger) is also statistically associated with increased serum IgE levels.

119.   In systemic lupus erythematosis, self antibodies are produced against:
   A. Double stranded DNA
   B. Single stranded DNA
   C. Transcription factors
   D. Histones
   E. All of the above

E is correct.
Antibodies to all of these are seldom found in a single patient, but cases are known in which antibodies to each component listed can be found. Interestingly, some of the transcription factors (e.g. Ku) were first identified by isolating the target of antibodies made by SLE patients.

120.   Superantigens:
   A. Bind to all members of a given Vβ family of T-cell receptor (TCR) variable regions
   B. Bind to the variable region of the TCRβ chain
   C. Act as mitogens for most B cells
   D. Are scientifically interesting but clinically unimportant
   E. Must be processed by macrophages (but not B cells) and presented to helper T cells

B is correct.
Superantigens bind to invariant sequences in the TCRβ variable region family and simultaneously to the MHC class II protein. Since these sequences vary with the family, stimulation is limited to the particular family(s) that have the relevant sequence. They stimulate only T cells since B cells do not have the relevant amino acid sequences. They do not require processing, indeed processing destroys their superantigen activity. Some superantigens are important bacterial exotoxins that cause significant pathology.

121. Farmer's lung would be treated with:
    A. Ibuprofen to suppress the inflammatory reaction
    B. Systemic corticosteroids
    C. Desensitization via intradermal injections of antigen
    D. IFN-γ to stimulate macrophages
    E. Chromlyn sodium

B is correct.
The immune response must be suppressed to prevent further lung injury.

For questions 122–125, match the lettered disease with the statement describing the immune pathology.

    A. Goodpasture's syndrome
    B. Allergic rhinitis
    C. Poison ivy reaction
    D. Systemic lupus erythematosis
    E. Arthus reaction

122. Systemic immune complex deposition.

E is correct.
The immune complexes are deposited in vascular beds of the kidney, lungs and (to a lesser extent) the joints. Complement fixation in these areas results in kidney and lung injury and joint pain.

123. Mediated by IgE.

B is correct.
IgE is the mediator of immediate hypersensitivity reactions of which hay fever (allergic rhinitis) is the most common example.

124. Mediated by antibody against basement membrane.

A is correct.
This is the prototypical type II reaction. The antibodies to basement membrane impair its function with subsequent kidney and lung failure.

125. Mediated by Th1 cells.

C is correct.
The delayed hypersensitivity reaction to poison ivy is a common example of contact dermatitis. Th1 cells are thought to be the delayed hypersensitivity T cells that mediate type IV reactions.

Autoimmunity

For questions 126–134, choose the single best answer.

126. HLA-B27 is a risk factor for which of the following autoimmune diseases?
    A. Lupus erythematosis
    B. Insulin-dependent diabetes mellitus
    C. Myasthenia gravis
    D. Multiple sclerosis
    E. Several arthritis-type diseases

E is correct.
B27 is most strongly associated with ankylosing spondylitis, but it is also found in higher than chance percentages in Reiter's disease and reactive arthritis (i.e. arthritis following infections such as *Yersinia*).

127. Tolerance to a particular antigen may be due to all of the following EXCEPT:
    A. Lack of Th cells for that antigen
    B. Overactive macrophages that completely degrade the antigen rather than expressing some on their surface
    C. High levels of antigen that block the antigen receptors on T and B cells
    D. Suppression of the response by Ts cells specific for that antigen
    E. Inability of the T and B cells to recognize that particular antigen

B is correct.
Macrophages are good at degrading antigens, but not that good. Lack of Th cells could be due to their deletion in the thymus. Loss of specific Ts cells in old age seems to be one reason why some elderly people become susceptible to autoimmune diseases.

128. Which of the following mechanisms is the most important in self-tolerance?
    A. Deletion of self-reactive clones of lymphocytes during their maturation in the central lymphoid organs
    B. Elimination of self-reactive Ts cells
    C. Continuous release of large amounts of self antigens into circulation
    D. Stimulation of Th1 cells to make cytokines that suppress IL-2 production
    E. Prevention of reactive lymphocytes from seeing stimulatory amounts of self antigen

A is correct.
Elimination of self-reactive Ts cells would tend to break self-tolerance. The others may contribute to some types of self-tolerance, but they are not the major explanation.

129. Which of the following mechanisms accounts for the relative ease of tolerance induction by deaggregated antigens?
    A. They usually induce Ts cells because they are presented by macrophages
    B. Antigen presenting cells have difficulty taking up and processing single chain proteins
    C. They are usually T independent antigens
    D. They overwhelm the antigen receptors on T cells producing high zone tolerance
    E. Serum proteases remove them so quickly that they do not have time to induce a response

B is correct.
Macrophages do not take up antigens smaller than 1 μm in diameter very efficiently. Thus, deaggregated antigens are less likely to be processed and presented in association with MHC class II proteins.

130. Which of the following is an example of an organ-specific autoimmune disease?
    A. Graves' disease
    B. Rheumatoid arthritis
    C. Goodpasture's syndrome
    D. Lupus erythematosis
    E. Sjögren's syndrome

A is correct.
Graves' disease is due to autoantibodies to the TSH receptors that stimulate thyroxin secretion. The other diseases are all systemic or multiorgan autoimmune diseases, e.g. Goodpasture's syndrome affects both the kidneys and the lungs.

131. Which of the following can result in autoimmunity?
    A. Oversuppression of suppressor cells
    B. Antigens similar or identical to self antigens are expressed on bacteria causing an infection
    C. Adult antigens are transferred across the placenta
    D. A patient undergoes chemotherapy for cancer
    E. A baby is born without a functional thymus

B is correct.
This is a method of bypassing lack of T helper cells. The other activities would tend to suppress the immune response, making autoimmunity less likely.

132.   An increased risk of developing insulin-dependent diabetes mellitus is associated with which of the following HLA alleles?
   A. DQ-3.2
   B. DR-3
   C. DR-4
   D. B-8
   E. B-27

A is correct.
The linkage was originally thought to be with DR-4. More recent analysis indicates that the incorrect association was due to linkage disequilibrium between DQ-3.2 and DR-4. DR-3 and DR-4 are associated with increased risk of rheumatoid arthritis; B-8 with myasthenia gravis; B-27 with ankylosing spondylitis.

133.   The inability to respond to self-antigens is called:
   A. Hyporesponsiveness
   B. Innate immunity
   C. Clonal selection
   D. Tolerance
   E. Primary immunity

D is correct.
Tolerance is the inability to respond to antigens to which other members of the species can mount an immune response. We are tolerant to our own tissues, whereas other people would often recognize them as foreign and produce a strong response.

134.   Which of the following is true of rheumatoid factors?
   A. They are autoantibodies to IgM
   B. They are antibody–collagen immune complexes
   C. They are autoantibodies to complement component C3b
   D. They are autoantibodies to IgG
   E. They are genes associated with an increased risk of developing rheumatoid arthritis

D is correct.
The antibodies to the Fc piece of IgG can be IgM, IgA or IgG. They are found in other conditions, so they are not diagnostic for rheumatoid arthritis.

Immunobiology of Cancer

For questions 135–142, choose the single best answer.

135.   Which of the following is characteristic of oncogenes?
   A. They induce development of most cancers
   B. They regulate the D–J rearrangement necessary for myeloma formation
   C. They probably originated from normal growth-regulating proteins
   D. They induce the target cell to secrete growth hormone which then stimulates continuous division of the cell
   E. They are derived from bacterial plasmids that give them drug resistance

C is correct.
Oncogenes normally produce necessary growth-inducing proteins. However, in cancers the control elements have been damaged such that they no longer respond to the normal signals that turn them off. Overproduction of the growth factors stimulates unregulated growth of the cells, i.e. cancer.

136.   An increase in which of the following would indicate recurrence of a liver cancer (hepatoma) that had been surgically removed two years previously?
   A. AFP (α-fetoprotein)
   B. Carcinoembryonic antigen
   C. IL-1
   D. Vasoactive intestinal peptide
   E. Substance P

A is correct.
Carcinoembryonic antigen is often elevated in cancers of the gastrointestinal and respiratory tracts. AFP is an embryonic antigen that is often elevated in hepatocarcinomas.

137.   Waldenstrom's macroglobulinemia is characterized by secretion of which of the following?
   A. Polyclonal IgM
   B. Monoclonal IgM
   C. Polyclonal IgG
   D. Monoclonal IgG
   E. IFN-γ

B is correct.
Myelomas secrete monoclonal antibodies. Waldenstrom's is a myeloma but does not carry the name because the symptoms produced are different from those produced by myelomas of the monomeric immunoglobulin classes.

138.   Which of the following cancers is the result of Epstein–Barr virus-induced translocation of an oncogene to the μ chain locus on chromosome 14?
   A. Thymoma
   B. Marek's disease
   C. Malignant melanoma
   D. Burkitt's lymphoma
   E. Hairy cell leukemia

D is correct.
The translocation is such that the signals that would normally induce IgM synthesis now result in production of the *c-myc* protein, a growth factor. Marek's disease (a chicken lymphoma) and hairy cell leukemia are both caused by viruses, but not E-B. The others are not known to be virally associated.

139.   Carcinoembryonic antigen is often elevated in people with which type of cancer?
   A. Bone
   B. Brain
   C. Liver
   D. Prostate
   E. Colon

E is correct.
CEA is an oncofetal antigen (an antigen that is normally present during embryogenesis and declines to almost undetectable levels shortly after birth, but increases during some types of cancer) that increases in about 35% of patients with colon or pancreatic cancer. α-Fetoprotein is another oncofetal antigen that can serve as a marker, in this case for hepatocellular carcinoma. It is elevated in 69% of patients with this cancer and has very few false positives.

140.   Which of the following cells are most specific for the cancer from which they were isolated?
   A. Macrophages
   B. PMNs
   C. TIL (tumor infiltrating lymphocytes)
   D. NK cells
   E. LAK cells

C is correct.
Macrophages, PMNs and NK cells are non-specific. Lymphokine activated killer cells derive from NK cells, therefore they are also non-specific.

141.   Which of the following have both cytotoxic and cytostatic activity?
   A. Macrophages
   B. PMNs
   C. TIL (tumor infiltrating lymphocytes)
   D. NK cells
   E. LAK cells

A is correct.
They are the only cells that have significant cytostatic activity, probably from secretion of prostaglandins. This is important because cancer is a balance between growth of the cancer cells and their destruction by host defenses. Anything that slows growth of the cancer may let the host defenses get ahead of growth and cause regression of the cancer.

142.   Which of the following has NOT been used to potentiate the immune system to attack cancer cells?
   A. Thymosin
   B. Monoclonal antibody
   C. IL-2
   D. TNF
   E. IFN

B is correct.
Monoclonal antibody has been used to treat cancers, but it acts directly on the cancers and/or opsonizes them for removal by ADCC. The others potentiate lymphocyte (immune system) responses, although thymosin has not been very successful.

Immunobiology of Transplantation

For questions 143 and 144, match the lettered blood type with the numbered statement.

A. A⁻
B. AB⁺
C. AB⁻
D. O⁺
E. O⁻

143.   People with which blood type are considered universal donors?

E is correct.
These erythrocytes lack A, B and D antigens, so the anti-A, anti-B and/or anti-D antibodies that occur in recipients with other blood types would have no target.

144.   People with which blood type are considered universal recipients?

B is correct.
Since these people have A, B and D antigens, they do not make antibodies to any of the antigens. Thus, they can accept any blood type without destroying the erythrocytes.

For questions 145–155, choose the single best answer.

145.   What is the term for a bone marrow transplant between identical twins?
   A. Syngeneic
   B. Autologous
   C. Allogeneic
   D. Heterogeneic

A is correct.
Identical twins are equivalent to an inbred strain of mice for which the term syngeneic was coined.

146.   A baby with blood type O⁺ has a mother who is type A⁻. A man with which of the following blood types could NOT be the father?
   A. A⁺
   B. B⁺
   C. O⁻
   D. O⁺

C is correct.
The father must be Rh⁺. The mother could be genotype AH (H is the genotype of type O), so she could have a baby with type O⁺ with a man who was AH, BH or HH.

147.   Kidney from a cadaver transplanted to a person of the same sex is termed:
   A. Syngeneic
   B. Autologous
   C. Allogeneic
   D. Heterogeneic

C is correct.
Allogeneic transplants are those between non-identical members of the same species. The fact that it came from a cadaver does not change that.

148.   Graft vs. host (GvH) disease is most likely to follow transplantation of which tissue?
   A. Heart
   B. Bone marrow
   C. Skin
   D. Kidney
   E. Pancreas

B is correct.
Bone marrow is the only tissue listed that contains numerous mature, immunocompetent T cells that are responsible for GvH disease.

149. Hemolytic disease of the newborn is classified as which type of tissue injury?
   A. Type I
   B. Type II
   C. Type III
   D. Type IV
   E. Combined types II and III

B is correct.
Type II is mediated by cytotoxic antibodies. Hemolytic disease of the newborn is due to destruction of the baby's erythrocytes by cytoxic antibodies. The fact that they are from the mother is irrelevant.

150. A kidney transplant from a parent to a same-sex child is termed:
   A. Syngeneic
   B. Autologous
   C. Allogeneic
   D. Heterogeneic

C is correct.
Half of the child's HLA antigens come from the other parent, so this is still considered an allograft.

151. Transfusion reactions that result in both intravascular and extravascular hemolysis of erythrocytes are due to which of the following?
   A. Anti-A antibodies
   B. Anti-B antibodies
   C. Anti-Rh antibodies
   D. Circulating immune complexes
   E. TNF-α

C is correct.
Extravascular hemolysis implies that IgG is involved. Blood groups A and B are determined by carbohydrate antigens that induce IgM. Rh is a protein antigen that induces IgG.

152. Which of the following is NOT involved in induction of anti-self antibodies?
   A. An injury that releases sequestered antigen
   B. Overcoming the lack of Th cells by having the self antigen associated with a bacterial protein that could act as a carrier
   C. Induction of Ts cells
   D. Blood transfusions
   E. Reactions induced by a foreign hapten, e.g. a drug binding to self proteins

C is correct.
Induction of Ts cells would tend to maintain tolerance.

153. Hyperacute rejection is caused by which of the following?
   A. Preformed antibody
   B. Presensitized CD4$^+$ T cells
   C. Presensitized CD8$^+$ T cells
   D. Mixed lymphocyte reaction

A is correct.
The preformed antibody comes from the patient having been exposed to the foreign MHC antigens previously, most commonly during a blood transfusion. Hyperacute rejection occurs within a few minutes of the transplant, which is faster than T cells are able to react. The MLR is the *in vitro* version of the mixed lymphocyte reaction.

154. The mixed lymphocyte response occurs when:
   A. Lymphocytes from two individuals with different MHC class I alleles are mixed.
   B. Lymphocytes from two individuals with different MHC class II alleles are mixed.
   C. Lymphocytes are mixed with stimulated antigen presenting cells from the same individual.
   D. Lymphocytes are incubated with a mixture of three cytokines, e.g. IL-2, IL-4 and IFNγ.
   E. A and D above.

B is correct.
The class II mismatch acts like class II antigen complexed with foreign antigen that a majority of Th cells can recognize. Class I mismatches stimulate an immune response, but it is comparable to that seen with normal antigen stimulation. Stimulated APCs and particularly some combinations of cytokines would stimulate lymphoproliferation but not at the levels of the mixed lymphocyte response.

155. The common blood typing done in most blood banks would identify a person without terminal fucosyl transferase and glactosyl transferase but with N-acetylglucosamine transferase as which blood type?
  A. Type A
  B. Type B
  C. Type AB
  D. Type O

D is correct.
This donor is unable to make the H substance, so he or she is actually a Bombay blood type. Even though the donor has the enzyme that would normally produce type A blood, there is no substrate for the enzyme. The test looks for antibodies to types A and B antigens. The donor would have both types, which is characteristic of type O blood.

Intervention in the Immune Response

For questions 156–166, choose the single best answer.

156. Immunopotentiating compounds that act as antigen depots include:
  A. Muramyl dipeptide
  B. Polynucleotides
  C. Aluminum hydroxide
  D. IFN-γ
  E. Lipopolysaccharide

C is correct.
Aluminum hydroxide (alum) is the most common adjuvant used in the United States. The others act by stimulating cells of the immune response.

157. Which of the following drugs acts by blocking transcription factors that are needed for IL-2 expression?
  A. Azathioprine
  B. Cyclophosphamide
  C. Cyclosporin A
  D. Prednisone
  E. FK506

C is correct.
FK506 also suppresses lymphokine function but via a different mechanism. The other factors act at different points in the immune response which is what makes 'triple therapy' with CsA, AZA and prednisone so effective in preventing graft rejection.

158. Which of the following immunosuppressive drugs acts as a competitive inhibitor in DNA synthesis?
  A. Azathioprine
  B. Cyclophosphamide
  C. Cyclosporin A
  D. Prednisone
  E. FK506

A is correct.
Azathioprine blocks all cell replication, not just that in the immune system. The other factors act at different points in the immune response which is what makes 'triple therapy' with CsA, AZA and prednisone so effective in preventing graft rejection.

159. Which of the following immunopotentiating drugs is routinely used in treatment of hairy cell leukemia?
  A. IL-2
  B. BCG
  C. Monoclonal antibody to leukemia antigens
  D. Thymosin
  E. IFN-α

E is correct.
Over 70% of patients with hairy cell leukemia *and* patients with chronic myeloid leukemia show complete or partial remission following treatment with this cytokine. None of the others has a dramatic effect on this disease.

160.   Which of the following drugs acts by inhibiting APC function, reducing MHC expression, and repressing cytotoxic T-cell generation?
   A.   Azathioprine
   B.   Cyclophosphamide
   C.   Cyclosporin A
   D.   Prednisone
   E.   FK506

D is correct.
Prednisone (the most commonly used form of cortisone) also interferes with leukocyte recirculation. Many of its effects on leukocytes are the opposite of the effects of IFNγ. The other factors act at different points in the immune response which is what makes 'triple therapy' with CsA, AZA, and prednisone so effective in preventing graft rejection.

161.   Antilymphocyte serum (ALS) suppresses graft rejection by:
   A.   Inducing T suppressor cells
   B.   Inhibiting the humoral immune response
   C.   Destroying passenger leukocytes in the transplanted tissue that would provoke rejection
   D.   Destroying recipient T cells
   E.   Destroying both T and B cells in the recipient

D is correct.
The ALS opsonizes the T cells but not B cells for removal by complement and phagocytes.

162.   A viral antigen isolated from a culture of yeast into which the viral gene had been inserted is used as the vaccine for which of the following?
   A.   Hepatitis B
   B.   AIDS
   C.   Mumps
   D.   Shingles
   E.   Influenza

A is correct.
Vaccines made from the surface antigen from hepatitis B provide effective protection to at-risk populations. The antigen from genetically engineered yeast is cleaner and cheaper than that isolated from the serum of infected patients.

163.   DPT vaccine is normally given:
   A.   In three doses at monthly intervals starting at 2–6 months of age
   B.   In one dose with adjuvant at 1 year of age
   C.   In three doses at weekly intervals starting at 12 months of age
   D.   In three doses at monthly intervals starting at 18 months of age
   E.   In two doses at 6 months and 12 months of age.

A is correct.
These diseases strike very young children, so it is important to protect them early. Booster shots are given at 15 months and 4 years. The Sabin polio vaccine is usually given concurrently with the DPT.

164.   Which of the following immunosuppressive drugs acts by cross-linking DNA?
   A.   Azathioprine
   B.   Cyclophosphamide
   C.   Cyclosporin A
   D.   Prednisone
   E.   FK506

B is correct.
Cyclophosphamide blocks all cell replication, so its effect is similar to that of azathioprine. It is commonly used in treating various autoimmune diseases.

165.   Infusion of immunoglobulin from a person who has had rubella into a pregnant woman who has been exposed to rubella is an example of which of the following?
   A. Active immunization
   B. Passive immunization
   C. Natural immunization
   D. Transfusion reaction

B is correct.
Passive immunity results from the transfer of immune lymphocytes or products of immune lymphocytes. Immunity is of short duration, lasting until the cells die or the soluble products are used up or degraded. This is in contrast to active immunity which results when antigen stimulates formation of memory cells that can respond to an infection so quickly that it is controlled before it becomes clinically effective.

166.   Which of following has been successfully treated with colony stimulating factors?
   A. Aplastic anemia
   B. Chronic graft rejection
   C. Chronic granulomatous disease
   D. Idiopathic thrombocytopenia
   E. Breast cancer

A is correct.
CSFs stimulate stem cells for both erythrocytes and leukocytes. They are most often used to speed recovery from bone marrow ablation during treatment for various cancers. However, they do not treat the cancer, but help the recovery from the treatment. They would probably aggravate graft rejection by stimulating production of more reactive leukocytes. CSFs would simply stimulate production of more defective phagocytes in CGD. Currently, there are no CSFs for platelets, which are the deficient cells in thrombocytopenia.

III.   GENERAL VIROLOGY

Virus Structure, Growth, Assay and Inactivation

For questions 167–172, choose the single best answer.

167.   Which of the following statements does NOT apply to virions?
  A. Virions are the basic units of all viruses
  B. Virions do not reproduce by division
  C. Virions must contain in their structure both DNA and RNA
  D. Virions may contain one or more enzymes
  E. Virions are obligate intracellular parasites

C is correct.
It is the only statement that does not apply to virions.

168.   A virion need not contain in its structure any other constituents than:
  A. Nucleic acid
  B. Protein
  C. DNA and RNA
  D. Nucleic acid and protein
  E. Lipid

D is correct.
The virions of naked viruses consist only of nucleic acid genomes and proteinaceous capsids. While enveloped viruses have an additional lipid covering, there is no virion which is made up of nucleic acid protein or lipid only. However, there are plant pathogens called viroids that are small, naked, circular RNA molecules, and mammalian pathogens called prions consisting of proteins only (see question 169 below).

169.   Prions are best described as:
  A. Proteinaceous infectious entities
  B. Typical viruses which occasionally cause terminal neurological disease
  C. Infectious entities consisting of naked circular RNA genomes
  D. Infectious agents causing disease in plants only
  E. A and B above

A is correct.
Prions, the etiological agents of the terminal CNS diseases CJD and Kuru in humans and scrapie in sheep are not typical viruses. They are believed to contain only protein in their structure and to originate from cellular genetic information.

170.   The capsids of all viruses carry out which of the following functions?
  A. Induce cell fusion
  B. Attach to host cells
  C. Induce virus neutralizing antibodies
  D. Protect genome nucleic acids from nucleases

D is correct.
Capsids protect nucleic acid genomes of all viruses. Induction of cell fusion is the function of a fusogenic protein found in the envelope of some enveloped viruses. Only naked viruses attach to host cells via their capsid proteins (see also answer to question 171 below).

171.   Virus neutralizing antibodies are likely to be directed at which of the following structural components of an enveloped virus?
   A. Capsid proteins
   B. Envelope glycoproteins
   C. Nucleic acid genome
   D. Envelope lipids
   E. All structural components

B is correct.
Neutralizing antibodies are directed at virion surface structures involved in attachment to host cells. These are glycoprotein spikes of enveloped viruses and capsid proteins of naked viruses. Antibodies to internal structures will not bind to intact virus particles or prevent them from infecting host cells. Lipids do not induce antibody formation.

172.   Which of the following statements is correct regarding enzymes in virus particles?
   A. By definition virus particles do not contain enzymes
   B. The virions of all viruses contain at least one enzyme
   C. Some viruses contain one or more enzymes in their virions
   D. The enzymes found in viruses are of host cell origin
   E. None of the above

C is correct.
The virions of several viruses contain one or a few enzymes such as polymerases and protein kinases. These are derived from viral genetic information.

For questions 173–177, match the viruses with the lettered characteristics.

   A. Bullet-shaped virions
   B. Diploid RNA genome
   C. Single-stranded DNA genome
   D. Presence of neuraminidase on virion surface
   E. Partially double-stranded circular DNA genome
   F. Double-stranded intact RNA genome
   G. Double-stranded linear DNA genome
   H. Double-stranded circular DNA genome

173.   Influenza virus.

D is correct.
Influenza viruses are characterized by neuraminidase and hemagglutinin spikes in their envelopes and segmented, (–)-sense, single-stranded RNA genomes.

174.   Hepatitis B virus.

E is correct.
Among DNA viruses, hepatitis B virus alone has a partially double-stranded circular DNA genome.

175.   Human T-cell leukemia virus.

B is correct.
Diploid RNA genomes are present only in human T-cell leukemia virus and other retroviruses.

176.   *Herpesvirus simiae.*

G is correct.
All herpesviruses have double-stranded linear DNA genomes.

177.   No animal virus.

F is correct.
No animal virus is known to contain intact double-stranded RNA. Members of the family Reoviridae contain double-stranded segmented RNA.
Guide to unmatched choices:
A: Bullet-shaped virions are characteristic of rabies virus and other rhabdoviruses.
C: Among known animal viruses, parvoviruses alone have single-stranded DNA genomes.
H: Only papillomaviruses and other papovaviruses contain double-stranded circular DNA genomes.

For questions 178–183, choose the single best answer.

178.   Some subgroups within virus families contain numerous serotypes. Serotype distinction is based on differences in:
    A. The antigenicity of virion surface proteins
    B. The nucleic acid characteristics
    C. Capsid symmetry
    D. Virion morphology
    E. All of the above

A is correct.
All members within a subgroup are very similar in all of the other characteristics. Unique antigens (epitopes) on virions define each serotype.

179.   For diagnosis of viral diseases by virus isolation, the medium most commonly used is:
    A. Embryonated eggs
    B. Organ cultures
    C. A suitable experimental animal
    D. An appropriate cell culture
    E. None of the above

D is correct.
Before the advent of cell cultures, embryonated eggs were commonly used. Organ cultures are impractical and unnecessary for the growth of most viruses. Experimental animals are expensive and of limited usefulness since most human viruses will not infect other animals.

180.   The medium commonly used to grow type A influenza virus for vaccine preparation is:
    A. Pigs
    B. Cell cultures of human origin
    C. 10-day-old embryonated eggs
    D. Organ cultures
    E. None of the above

C is correct.
Influenza virus for vaccine production is grown in embryonated eggs even though it will also grow in cell cultures. Organ cultures are inappropriate (see question 179 above). Although type A influenza virus will infect other animals, practical considerations preclude the use of animals for the production of large quantities of virus.

181.   Suckling mice inoculation is the method of choice for the primary isolation of:
    A. Coxsackie viruses
    B. Polioviruses
    C. Echoviruses
    D. All enteroviruses
    E. None of the above

A is correct.
Some coxsackie viruses will not grow in any medium other than suckling mice for which all coxsackie viruses are highly virulent. The other enteroviruses, namely echoviruses and polio-viruses, grow readily in cell cultures of primate origin.

182.   None of the following viruses of humans can be grown *in vitro* EXCEPT:
   A. Papillomaviruses
   B. Epstein–Barr virus
   C. Norwalk agents
   D. Hepatitis virus types B and C
   E. Hepatitis virus type E

B is correct.
Epstein–Barr virus is the exception because it can be grown in primate B-cell cultures. The other viruses cannot be cultivated *in vitro*.

183.   Cell cultures derived from various mammalian species can be used for the isolation of:
   A. Human coronavirus
   B. Chicken pox virus
   C. Herpes simplex virus
   D. Human T-cell leukemia virus

C is correct.
Herpes simplex virus will grow in cell cultures of human and non-human origin. Human coronaviruses are fastidious; some of them require organ cultures of human embryonic trachea for growth *in vitro*. Chicken pox virus and human T-cell leukemia virus require appropriate human-derived cell cultures for growth *in vitro*.

For questions 184–186, match the lettered virus with its numbered receptor on the host cell surface.

   A. Acetylcholine receptor
   B. Blood group antigen P
   C. Heparan sulfate
   D. Intercellular adhesion molecule-1 (ICAM-1)
   E. Complement C3d receptor

184.   Human rhinovirus.

D is correct.

185.   Parvovirus.

B is correct.

186.   Epstein–Barr virus.

E is correct.
Guide to unmatched choices:
A: Acetylcholine receptor is used by rabies virus to infect neurons.
C: The cell surface molecule heparan sulfate is believed to be the receptor for herpes simplex virus.

For questions 187–190, choose the single best answer.

187.   The inability of a virus to infect certain tissues in a host could be explained by:
   A. The absence in tissue cells of virus-specific receptors
   B. The absence in tissue cells of transcription factors needed for viral gene expression
   C. Either of the above
   D. Neither of the above

C is correct.
In addition to specific receptors which all viruses require to enter their host cells, some viruses require tissue-specific transcription factors for their replication.

188.   To measure the total number of virus particles in a purified preparation of any virus, the method of choice is:
   A. Pock assay
   B. Plaque assay
   C. Electron microscopic assay
   D. Hemagglutination assay
   E. Any of the above

C is correct.
Plaque assay and pock assay quantify infectious virus particles only. Hemagglutination assay measures the approximate total number of virus particles but is limited by its applicability only to viruses which agglutinate red blood cells.

189. Embryonated eggs are used to assay viruses using the procedure known as:
    A. Plaque assay
    B. Pock assay
    C. Lethal dose 50 assay (LD50 assay)
    D. Hemagglutination assay
    E. None of the above

B is correct.
Pock assay measures the number of foci of infection (pocks) in the chorioallantoic membrane. Plaque assay uses monolayer cultures of cells, LD50 assay employs experimental animals and hemagglutination assay requires red blood cells.

190. All of the following assays measure infective virions EXCEPT:
    A. LD50 assay
    B. Hemagglutination assay
    C. Pock assay
    D. Plaque assay

B is correct.
Hemagglutination assay measures the approximate total number of hemagglutinating virus particles, not just infectious virus particles in a virus preparation.

For questions 191–195, choose whether the statement is true or false.

191. Poliovirus is more easily inactivated by environmental heat than herpes simplex virus.

False.
Herpes simplex virus is enveloped whereas poliovirus is naked. Heat destroys the integrity of viral envelopes by increasing the fluidity of envelope lipids. Without an intact envelope, herpes and other enveloped viruses cannot infect efficiently. The coats of naked viruses such as poliovirus consisting of only protein are relatively more heat resistant.

192. Powerful oxidizing agents such as Clorox (hypochlorite) inactivate all viruses and virus-like agents.

True.
Oxidizing agents denature all proteins and nucleic acids. Therefore, all viruses and virus-like proteinaceous infectious entities (prions) are inactivated by such agents.

193. The inactivation of viruses by ionizing radiation is solely due to the breakage of their genome nucleic acid strands.

False.
In addition to strand scission, ionizing radiation generates reactive OH^- radicals which oxidize and denature amino acids in proteins and bases in nucleic acids.

194. Formaldehyde-treated viruses are suitable for immunization because formaldehyde reduces the virulence of viruses without inactivating them.

False.
Formaldehyde inactivates viruses primarily by reacting with NH_2 groups in nucleic acids and denaturing them. Formaldehyde also reacts with the NH_2 groups of proteins, but apparently does not alter the immunogenicity of such proteins.

195. Poliovirus cannot multiply in chicken cells because chicken cells lack the transcription factor necessary for poliovirus replication.

False.
The lack of poliovirus-specific receptor on chicken cells is the explanation. The evidence for this conclusion is that poliovirus RNA alone can cause productive infection in chicken cells. Poliovirus RNA is an infectious nucleic acid.

Viral Replication

For questions 196–202, choose the single best answer.

196.   All of the following statements about infectious viral nucleic acids are correct EXCEPT:
   A. They are relatively more heat resistant than virions
   B. They are far less efficient than virions in initiating infection
   C. They are not inactivated by antiviral antibodies
   D. They are inactivated by nucleases
   E. They are taken up by cells via nucleic acid-specific receptors

E is correct.
Infectious viral nucleic acids are taken up by cells non-specifically, not via receptors. The other responses all apply to infectious nucleic acids.

197.   If a virus nucleic acid genome alone can infect cells and produce progeny, one may conclude that:
   A. The virus has a (+)-sense RNA genome
   B. The viral genome replicates in the nucleus
   C. The viral genome replicates in the cytoplasm
   D. The viral genome either serves as mRNA or can be transcribed by pre-existing cellular enzymes
   E. None of the above

D is correct.
In order for a naked viral genome to be an infectious nucleic acid it must produce in the host cell, mRNA for viral-specific proteins. The (+)-sense RNA genomes of group 1 RNA viruses (picorna-, calici-, flavi-, toga- and corona-) accomplish this by serving also as mRNA, and the DNA viral genomes replicating in the nucleus (parvo-, papova-, adeno- and herpes-) by using cellular RNA polymerase to produce virus-specific mRNA.

198.   All of the following viruses contain infectious nucleic acid genomes EXCEPT:
   A. Rhabdovirus
   B. Picornavirus
   C. Herpesvirus
   D. Adenovirus
   E. Coronavirus

A is correct.
Rhabdovirus RNA genome is (–)-sense, cannot serve as mRNA and therefore cannot be an infectious viral RNA. The RNA genomes of picornavirus and coronavirus are (+)-sense and serve as mRNA whereas the DNA genomes of herpesvirus and adenovirus are transcribed by cellular RNA polymerase. These four genomes are therefore infectious nucleic acids.

199.   If the nucleic acid genome alone of a virus infects cells and produces progeny, it is likely that:
   A. The virus does not contain a polymerase in its virions
   B. The virus has a (+)-sense RNA genome
   C. The viral genome replicates in the nucleus
   D. The viral genome is transcribed by cellular RNA polymerase II
   E. All of the above

A is correct.
The presence of a polymerase in the virion almost always correlates with a non-infectious nucleic acid genome. The only known exception is hepatitis B virus which contains a polymerase as well as an infectious nucleic acid (DNA) genome. Responses B and C are applicable to some but not all infectious nucleic acid genomes since only some such genomes are (+)-sense RNA or replicate in the nucleus.

200.   Papovavirus replication strategy includes all of the following EXCEPT:
   A. Use of cellular polymerases for genome transcription and replication
   B. Use of self-annealing 3'-terminus of genome as primer for DNA synthesis
   C. Bidirectional semi-conservative replication starting from a specific origin
   D. Unwinding of supercoiled circular DNA by an early viral gene product
   E. Replication in the cell nucleus

B is correct.
Papovavirus genome is supercoiled circular double stranded DNA. Replication strategy involves transcription of an early gene (T antigen) by cellular RNA polymerase, unwinding of the supercoiled DNA by T antigen and bidirectional semi-conservative replication by cellular DNA polymerase. Use of self annealing 3'-terminus of the genome as the primer for DNA synthesis is a strategy employed by the single-stranded DNA genome of parvoviruses.

201.   An RNA intermediate is involved in the replication of:
   A. Parvovirus
   B. Papovavirus
   C. Hepadnavirus
   D. Adenovirus
   E. Herpesvirus

C is correct.
All of the choices are DNA viruses. The only DNA virus which replicates its genome via an RNA intermediate is hepadnavirus (hepatitis B). First, cellular RNA polymerase II transcribes the (−) strand of the viral genome into a (+)-sense RNA intermediate (and virus-specific mRNAs). Then, a virus-specific DNA polymerase reverse transcribes the (+)-sense RNA into progeny DNA.

202.   Aplastic crisis in sickle-cell patients due to parvovirus B-19 infection results directly from:
   A. Viral replication in actively dividing red blood cell progenitors
   B. Viral replication in mature red blood cells
   C. Viral replication in the cellular nucleus
   D. Inability of the virus to stimulate DNA synthesis in host cells
   E. Use of cellular polymerases for viral genome replication and transcription

A is correct.
Blood group antigen P is the receptor for parvovirus B-19. Only dividing red blood cell progenitors can provide all of the requirements for parvovirus B-19 gene expression and genome replication, and killing of these cells by the virus leads to aplastic crisis in sickle-cell patients. Choice B is therefore incorrect. The other choices are true statements about parvovirus replication but are not directly responsible for aplastic crisis.

For questions 203–205, match the numbered viruses with the lettered statements.

   A. Genome RNA serves also as mRNA
   B. Viral mRNA is transcribed by cellular RNA polymerase II
   C. Viral mRNA cap structures are pirated from nascent cellular mRNA
   D. Viral mRNA becomes part of progeny viral genome RNA

203.   Flaviviridae (Class 1 RNA viruses).

A is correct.
It is characteristic of all Group 1 RNA viruses that their (+)-sense RNA genomes also serve as mRNA. Picorna-, flavi-, toga- and coronaviruses are included in this group.

204.   Reoviridae (Class 5 RNA viruses).

D is correct.
Each segment of reovirus genome specifies a (+)-sense RNA which first serves as mRNA, then as a template for (−) RNA, and with the latter it forms a progeny double-stranded genome segment.

205.   Orthomyxoviridae (Class 3 RNA viruses).

C is correct.
Orthomyxoviruses are the only viruses known which use cap structures pirated from nascent cellular mRNA as primers for synthesis of their mRNAs.
Guide to unmatched choice:
B: Statement B is true of all DNA viruses replicating in the cellular nucleus, hepadnaviruses which replicate partially in the nucleus and partially in the cytoplasm, and all retroviruses.

For questions 206–209, choose the single best answer.

206.   RNA-dependent RNA polymerases which replicate viral RNA genomes are NOT:
   A. Contained in the virions of all RNA viruses
   B. Specified by the genomes of RNA viruses
   C. Involved in the synthesis of viral mRNA as well as genome RNA
   D. Potentially useful targets for chemotherapy

A is correct.
The genomes of all RNA viruses except retroviruses specify and are copied by RNA-dependent RNA polymerases. All except class I RNA viruses package these enzymes in their virions. All other choices correctly describe these enzymes.

207.   Which of the following pairs of viruses uses a cellular polymerase for genome transcription but not for genome replication?
   A. Papovavirus and adenovirus
   B. Herpesvirus and papovavirus
   C. Adenovirus and herpesvirus
   D. Parvovirus and papovavirus
   E. None of the above

C is correct.
Adenoviruses and herpesviruses, like all DNA viruses which replicate in the nucleus, use cellular RNA polymerase II for genome transcription. However, unlike parvoviruses and papovaviruses, they use a virally specified DNA polymerase for genome replication.

208.   If protein synthesis is inhibited in host cells infected with poliovirus or herpes simplex virus (HSV), virus-specific mRNA synthesis will not be initiated in:
   A. HSV-infected cells only
   B. Poliovirus-infected cells only
   C. Both of the above
   D. Neither of the above

B is correct.
Before poliovirus-specific mRNA can be synthesized in infected cells, the RNA polymerase which copies the poliovirus genome must be produced by translation of the (+)-sense RNA genome. Cellular protein synthesis inhibitors prevent synthesis of this enzyme and poliovirus-specific mRNA synthesis will not occur. Cellular RNA polymerase II produces herpes simplex virus-specific mRNA, so transcription of early viral genes by pre-existing RNA polymerase II will not be affected by inhibition of cellular protein synthesis.

209. Inhibition of host cellular transcription will arrest the replication of:
   A. Picornaviruses and paramyxoviruses
   B. Arenaviruses and bunyaviruses
   C. Orthomyxoviruses and retroviruses
   D. Togaviruses and rhabdoviruses
   E. All DNA viruses but no RNA virus

C is correct.
Among viruses with RNA genomes, orthomyxoviruses and retroviruses alone depend on host cellular transcription for their replication. All other RNA viruses replicate solely in the cytoplasm and use only virus-specific polymerases (RNA-dependent RNA polymerases) for their replication. These enzymes are not inhibited by agents which block transcription of DNA. E is partially correct in that such agents will arrest transcription of viral DNA, and therefore inhibit replication of all DNA viruses.

Viral Transmission and Viral Persistence

For questions 210–228, choose the single best answer.

210. An example of a human virus which is transmitted vertically as well as horizontally is:
   A. Rhinovirus
   B. Rubella virus
   C. Coronavirus
   D. Rotavirus
   E. Adenovirus

B is correct.
Rubella virus can be transmitted horizontally via aerosolized respiratory secretions and vertically by placental transfer.

211. Congenital infection is a mechanism in the transmission of:
   A. Human immunodeficiency virus
   B. Cytomegalovirus
   C. Rubella virus
   D. Hepatitis B virus
   E. All of the above viruses

E is correct.
All of these viruses are known to be transmitted vertically from mother to offspring. Other viruses in this group include chicken pox virus, herpes simplex virus and coxsackie B virus.

212. An example of a human virus which can naturally infect other species is:
   A. Type A influenza virus
   B. Measles virus
   C. Smallpox virus
   D. Chicken pox virus
   E. Hepatitis B virus

A is correct.
Type A influenza virus infects not only humans but some other mammals and several species of birds under natural conditions. Humans are the only natural hosts for all of the other viruses listed.

213. Which of the following is NOT a true statement about arboviruses causing human disease?
   A. All of them have RNA genomes
   B. Arthropods are both vectors and hosts for these viruses
   C. Encephalitis and hemorrhagic fevers are the most serious arboviral diseases
   D. They are known to be transmitted between humans by person-to-person contact

D is correct.
The arthropod vector is essential for the transmission of arboviruses between their hosts. All of the other responses are true statements about arboviruses.

214.   Which of the following hosts are necessary and sufficient for the maintenance of arboviruses in nature?
   A. Birds and lower mammals
   B. Arthropods
   C. Humans
   D. Higher mammals
   E. Arthropods, birds and lower mammals

E is correct.
Birds and lower mammals amplify arboviral populations and arthropods transmit arboviruses between these hosts. Higher mammals and humans are considered to be accidental hosts, not essential for the maintenance of arboviruses in nature.

215.   Which of the following statements is NOT true about Dengue virus?
   A. It is biologically related to yellow fever
   B. It causes hemorrhagic fever
   C. Immune complexes are involved in disease causation
   D. Transmission is by mosquito vectors
   E. Humans cannot be the source of infection of other humans

E is correct.
It is the only statement that does not apply to Dengue virus. See also the answer to question 216 below.

216.   Which of the following is a human virus that belongs to a family consisting mostly of arthropod-borne zoonotic viruses?
   A. Dengue virus
   B. St. Louis encephalitis virus
   C. California encephalitis virus
   D. Colorado tick fever virus
   E. Rubella virus

E is correct.
Rubella virus, a human virus maintained in nature exclusively by human-to-human transmission, belongs to the family *Togaviridae*, which consists predominantly of arthropod-borne zoonotic viruses. All other viruses listed are arthropod-borne zoonotic viruses which cause disease in humans as well. Dengue virus, however, can maintain itself outside its zoonotic natural hosts by human-to-human transmission in urban areas where the mosquito vector of this virus is able to breed.

217.   Which of the following statements about rodent-borne viruses causing human disease is NOT true?
   A. Lymphocytic choriomeningitis virus is an example of such a virus
   B. They include viruses causing deadly hemorrhagic fevers
   C. Human-to-human transmission resulting from contact with infectious material occurs with some of these viruses
   D. Mosquitoes are usually involved in rodent-to-human transmission

D is correct.
Rodent-to-human transmission is via rodent excreta, not by mosquitoes or other vectors. All other responses are true statements about rodent-borne viruses causing human disease.

218.   Examples of rodent-borne viruses causing hemorrhagic fevers are all of the following EXCEPT:
   A. Hantavirus of Korea
   B. Yellow fever virus and Dengue virus of tropical and subtropical regions
   C. Junin virus and Machupo virus of South America
   D. Lassa fever virus of West Africa

D is correct.
Even though all of the above viruses cause hemorrhagic fevers, yellow fever virus and Dengue virus are arboviruses (mosquito-borne, not rodent-borne viruses).

219.   Which of the following is NOT a true statement about subclinical viral infections?
- A. Viruses most commonly produce subclinical infections
- B. The virus does not multiply in the tissues of a subclinically infected host
- C. The host is likely to develop specific immunity to reinfection with the same virus
- D. The virus may remain latent in the host following a subclinical infection

B is correct.
During subclinical infections there is limited virus replication in host cells so that the immune system is stimulated, but not enough host cells are destroyed to cause clinical disease.

220.   The factors which predict that an effective vaccine can be developed for the eradication of a human virus include all of the following EXCEPT:
- A. The existence of only a single serotype of the virus
- B. The absence of carriers
- C. The absence of non-human hosts for the virus
- D. Extreme contagiousness of the virus

D is correct.
Contagiousness has no bearing on eradication through the vaccination approach. The existence of only a single serotype makes it possible to develop an effective vaccine. The absence of carriers and non-human hosts for the virus predicts that eradication through vaccination will be feasible.

221.   Persistence of viruses in the host cell is facilitated by all of the following attributes EXCEPT:
- A. Antigenic variability
- B. Ability to cause latent infection
- C. Ability to multiply in macrophages without killing them
- D. Ability to inhibit immune responses
- E. Extreme virulence

E is correct.
A virus is unlikely to persist in hosts for which it has high virulence. The other attributes aid viral persistence.

222.   Persistence of human immunodeficiency virus (HIV) in the host is facilitated by:
- A. Latent infection of helper T cells
- B. Antigenic variability
- C. Multiplication in macrophages without killing them for long periods
- D. Virus-induced immunosuppression
- E. All of the above

E is correct.
HIV uses a variety of mechanisms known to aid viruses in their persistence.

223.   Which of the following is NOT a characteristic of all slow viral diseases?
- A. Long incubation period (years)
- B. Rare incidence
- C. CNS involvement
- D. Irreversibility (terminality)
- E. Amyloid plaques in the brain

E is correct.
The sponge-like appearance of the gray matter and amyloid plaques are characteristics of slow viral disease caused by prions but not by typical viruses.

224.   All of the following are slow viral diseases caused by prions EXCEPT:
- A. Creutzfeldt–Jacob disease (CJD)
- B. Systemic sclerosing panencephalitis (SSPE)
- C. Kuru
- D. Bovine spongiform encephalopathy (BSE)
- E. Scrapie

B is correct.
Of the diseases listed, SSPE alone is caused by a conventional virus, namely measles virus.
All of the others are prion diseases. Progressive multifocal leukoencephalopathy (PML) caused by the papovavirus JC virus is the other slow viral disease due to a conventional virus.

225. The slow viral disease resulting from immunosuppression is:
    A. Systemic sclerosing panencephalitis (SSPE)
    B. Progressive multifocal leukoencephalopathy (PML)
    C. Kuru
    D. Creutzfeldt–Jacob disease (CJD)
    E. Scrapie

B is correct.
PML caused by JC virus, a papovavirus, is the only known slow viral disease which occurs in immunodeficient or immunosuppressed patients. Kuru, CJD and scrapie are believed to be caused by prions which do not induce an immune response. Immunosuppression has no effect on the incidence or course of prion diseases.

226. Early childhood measles is a risk factor for the development of the slow viral disease:
    A. Progressive multifocal leukoencephalopathy (PML)
    B. Systemic sclerosing panencephalitis (SSPE)
    C. Creutzfeldt–Jacob disease (CJD)
    D. Kuru
    E. Scrapie

B is correct.
SSPE which usually occurs in adolescents is caused by the persistence of measles virus in a rare host. The incidence of SSPE is higher among children contracting measles before age 2 years.

227. Characteristics of the agent of Creutzfeldt–Jacob disease (CJD) include all of the following EXCEPT:
    A. A nucleic acid genome
    B. Lack of virion-like structure
    C. Lack of antigenicity
    D. Resistance to formaldehyde
    E. Endogenous origin

A is correct.
The agents of CJD, Kuru and scrapie are prions which are proteinaceous infectious entities lacking a nucleic acid genome, hence they have no virion-like structure. Prion protein originates as a (modified) host gene product (endogenous) and therefore lacks antigenicity. Prions can be transmitted between hosts (via surgical instruments, for instance) and are highly resistant to several physical and chemical agents including formaldehyde and phenol which inactivate typical viruses.

228. To disinfect a surface contaminated with prions all of the following agents will be ineffective EXCEPT:
    A. UV light
    B. X-rays
    C. Clorox (hypochlorite)
    D. Phenol
    E. Formaldehyde

C is correct.
Prions are inactivated by powerful oxidizing agents such as hypochlorite and by autoclaving. UV light and X-rays are directed primarily at nucleic acids which prions lack.

Antiviral Immune Responses

For questions 229–237, choose the single best answer.

229. If a virus spreads by inducing fusion of infected cells with susceptible cells, its dissemination in the patient cannot be halted by:
    A. Cytotoxic T cell-mediated cell killing
    B. Natural killer (NK) cell-mediated cell killing
    C. Neutralization by specific antibodies
    D. Antibody-dependent, complement-mediated cell lysis
    E. Any of the above mechanisms

C is correct.
Virus neutralization by antibodies occurs in tissue fluids. Cell-to-cell spread of a virus by fusion protects the virions from contact with antibodies. On the other hand, all of the other mechanisms are involved in the elimination of infected cells, and could therefore be effective in halting the spread of the virus in question.

230. The antiviral defense component that is targeted to virus-specific intracellur events is:
A. Interferon
B. Antiviral antibody
C. Macrophage
D. Cytotoxic T cell
E. NK cell

A is correct.
Interferon is the only component of the host defense system that arrests viral replication by targeting virus-specific translation or other intracellular events necessary for viral replication.

231. Non-specific mechanisms of antiviral host defense include:
A. Antibodies
B. Complement and interferon
C. Cytotoxic T cells
D. NK cells and macrophages
E. B and D above

E is correct.
Complement, interferon, NK cells and macrophages are the major components of non-specific antiviral host defense which acts against a variety of viruses. Cytotoxic T lymphocytes and antiviral antibodies are virus-specific.

232. Augmented immune response due to reinfection with a virus is mediated by:
A. Antibodies
B. NK cells and macrophages
C. Cytotoxic T cells
D. Interferon and complement
E. A and C above

E is correct.
Only specific immune responses mediated by antibodies and cytotoxic T cells are augmented during reinfection. The reason for enhanced secondary response is the presence of a memory cell population capable of forming a larger number of antibody-producing B cells (plasma cells) and cytotoxic T cells in reinfection than in primary infection. Reinfection does not enhance non-specific defense mechanisms.

233. The effector cells in antiviral host defense due to antibody-dependent cellular cytotoxicity (ADCC) are:
A. Killer (K) cells
B. Macrophages
C. K cells or macrophages
D. Cytotoxic T lymphocytes (CTLs)
E. Plasma cells

C is correct.
Both K cells, a subset of NK cells, and macrophages may participate in the elimination of antibody coated virus-infected cells by ADCC. Via the Fc receptor on their surface, the effector cells attach to the Fc portion of the antibody coating the target cells before killing them. Neither CTLs nor plasma cells are the effector cells in ADCC.

234. If a virus is able to inhibit the expression of MHC-1 on infected cell surfaces, such cells will NOT be destroyed by:
A. $CD4^+$ CTLs
B. $CD8^+$ CTLs
C. NK cells
D. Macrophages
E. Complement-mediated lysis

B is correct.
CTLs which are predominantly $CD8^+$ recognize only viral epitopes complexed with MHC-1 and presented on cell surfaces; their target recognition is MHC-1 restricted. Some viruses evade CTL action by preventing MHC-1 expression on cell surfaces. $CD4^+$ CTLs are MHC-II restricted and not commonly found.

235. The term virus neutralization means:
A. Elimination of antibody-attached virions by phagocytosis
B. Prevention of virus infection of cultured cells by antiviral antibody
C. Elimination of virus infected cells by antibody complement-mediated cell lysis
D. Elimination of virus-infected cells by ADCC
E. All of the above

B is correct.
This term specifically refers to inactivation of viral particles by specific antibody so that cultured cells cannot be affected.

236.   The role of antibodies in defense against viral diseases is best described by which of the following statements?

   A. Relatively less important than CTLs in preventing first infection
   B. More important than CTLs in recovery from most viral infections
   C. As important as CTLs in preventing as well as curing viral infections
   D. Of primary importance in preventing viral infections but less important than CTLs in recovery from most viral infections

D is correct.

Antiviral defense consists of preventing infection and eliminating infected cells. Antibodies in tissue fluids are of primary importance in preventing infection of cells. However, once infection has occurred, CTLs appear to be more important than antibodies in eliminating infected cells. The evidence for this view is that children with deficient antibody responses and normal CTL responses recover from most viral infections. Exceptions are certain enteroviral infections which persist in individuals with defective antibody responses even though they have normal T-cell responses.

237.   Upon contracting measles, tuberculin-positive individuals become tuberculin-negative. This indicates that:

   A. Measles virus is immunosuppressive
   B. Measles rash masks tuberculin reaction
   C. Measles virus inhibits IgE-mediated responses
   D. Tuberculin reaction cannot be observed in virus-infected patients in general
   E. All of the above

A is correct.

Tuberculin reaction is a manifestation of delayed type hypersensitivity (DHS) to a protein produced by the tubercle bacillus. DHS in turn is an aspect of cell-mediated immune response. Measles virus suppresses the immune response transiently and thereby blocks the tuberculin reaction. Any virus which inhibits T helper cell-responses will produce this effect. For this reason, the tuberculin reaction is absent or diminished in HIV-infected TB patients.

Viral Genetics

For questions 238–244, choose the single best answer.

238.   The genetic mechanism by which new pandemic strains of influenza virus arise is best described as:

   A. Complementation
   B. Mutation
   C. Recombination
   D. Genome segment reassortment
   E. Phenotypic mixing

D is correct.

Type A influenza virus undergoes constant minor genetic changes in its virulence genes (hemagglutin and neuraminidase genes) through mutations and sporadic major changes in these genes through genome segment reassortment. A major change in virulence leads to pandemics (world-wide epidemics).

239.   All viruses undergo genetic variation by:

   A. Recombination
   B. Mutation
   C. Genome segment reassortment
   D. Complementation
   E. All of the above mechanisms

B is correct.

All genomes are susceptible to random mutational change. Recombination is exhibited readily by DNA viral genomes and rarely by some intact RNA viral genomes. Genome segment reassortment is restricted to RNA viruses with segmented genomes. Complementation is a non-genetic phenomenon.

240.   A viral mutant arising in a patient will be able to
replace the parent if the mutation:
  A. Blocks neutralization by antibodies
  B. Occurs in the virulence gene of the virus
  C. Occurs in a virion surface protein
  D. Affects the rate of viral genome replication
  E. Is described by any of the above

A is correct.
As virus neutralizing antibodies eliminate the
parental virus type, mutants resisting neutralization by antibodies survive and replace the
parent. Mutations described by the other
responses do not imply that the mutants will have
a selective advantage over the parent.

241.   The major mechanism by which HIV genetic variants
arise in patients is:
  A. Recombination
  B. Genome segment reassortment
  C. Mutation
  D. Complementation
  E. None of the above

C is correct.
HIV replication involves two enzymes, i.e. virion
reverse transcriptase and host RNA polymerase
II. Neither enzyme has an editing function.
Therefore, occasional misincorporation of nucleo-
tides by these enzymes remains uncorrected. This
results in a high rate of mutation and genetic variation. Another mechanism mediating genetic
change in HIV is recombination between proviral
DNA molecules.

242.   A candidate attenuated viral vaccine is least likely to
revert to virulence if it is:
  A. A single point mutant
  B. A multiple point mutant
  C. A deletion mutant
  D. Deficient in virulence
  E. Any of the above

C is correct.
Deletion mutants lack a segment of the genome
and therefore cannot revert. (No viral vaccine
consisting of a deletion mutant is available as yet.)
Single point mutants will revert with relatively
high frequency. Multiple point mutants will also
revert even though at extremely low frequency as
evidenced by the attenuated (oral) poliovirus
vaccine. D cannot be the answer since an
attenuated virus is deficient in virulence by definition.

243.   All of the following statements describe
complementation by viruses EXCEPT:
  A. Occurs between two viral mutants which are
      defective in different genes
  B. Allows two non-viable mutants to reproduce
      themselves
  C. Occurs between mutants of the same virus or closely
      related viruses only
  D. Does not involve genetic recombination
  E. Involves genetic variation

E is correct.
Complementation is a non-genetic phenomenon
whereby the defective gene product of one virus is
replaced with the non-defective gene product of a
closely related, co-infecting virus. Both viruses
can be defective provided that the defect is in
different genes.

244.   When two unrelated enveloped viruses replicate
simultaneously in a host cell, the nucleocapsid of one virus
may accept the envelope specified by the other virus. This is
an example of:
  A. Complementation
  B. Phenotypic masking
  C. Genetic recombination
  D. Pseudo-virion formation
  E. All of the above

D is correct.
Pseudovirions are formed when the nucleocapsid
of one virus is enclosed in the envelope specified
by a different virus. Phenotypic masking occurs
when the progeny genomes of a naked virus
accept the capsid specified by a closely related co-
infecting virus. In genetic recombination,
genomes with identical or closely related
sequences base pair and exchange parts via
breakage and reunion as exemplified by DNA
viruses.

IV.   CLINICAL VIROLOGY

Enteric Viruses and Hepatitis Viruses

For questions 245–261, choose the single best answer.

245.   Which of the following viruses does NOT enter the host through intestinal epithelium?
   A. Coxsackie virus
   B. Echovirus
   C. Measles virus
   D. Rotavirus
   E. Norwalk agents

C is correct.
The exception is measles virus which enters via respiratory epithelium only.

246.   Intestinal disease is often caused by all of the following viruses EXCEPT:
   A. Norwalk agents
   B. Rotavirus
   C. Adenovirus
   D. Coronavirus
   E. Coxsackie virus

E is correct.
All of the listed viruses EXCEPT coxsackie virus cause diarrhea. Even though coxsackie virus enters the host through the intestinal tract it does not usually cause intestinal illness.

247.   Both respiratory and intestinal illness may be caused by:
   A. Adenovirus
   B. Coronavirus
   C. Poliovirus
   D. Echovirus
   E. A, B and D above

E is correct.
Adenovirus and coronavirus are respiratory viruses, but some serotypes of each cause intestinal illness. Echovirus may cause diarrhea in children and cold-like symptoms. Although poliovirus infects and replicates in the intestinal epithelium, like coxsackie virus, it does not cause intestinal disease.

248.   Examples of viruses causing intestinal as well as CNS infections are:
   A. Enterovirus subgroup of picornaviruses
   B. Rotaviruses and Norwalk agents
   C. Coronaviruses and adenoviruses
   D. Astroviruses and pestiviruses
   E. None of the above viruses

A is correct.
The enterovirus subgroup consists of polioviruses, coxsackie viruses and echoviruses, all of which enter the host through the intestinal tract and cause CNS infections. None of the other groups of viruses causes CNS infections. Astroviruses and pestiviruses are as yet poorly characterized RNA viruses causing diarrhea in humans.

249.   The illness which often results from infection with polioviruses, coxsackie viruses and echoviruses is:
   A. Common cold
   B. Herpangina
   C. Pleurodynia
   D. Hand, foot and mouth disease
   E. Asceptic meningitis

E is correct.
All three members of the enterovirus subgroup cause asceptic meningitis. Common cold-like symptoms are produced by coxsackie and echoviruses but not by polioviruses. Herpangina (throat lesions), pleurodynia (chest and abdominal pain) and hand, foot and mouth disease are all caused by coxsackie viruses.

250.   Which of the following viruses can cause heart disease in newborns as well as in adults?
  A. Coxsackie A virus
  B. Coxsackie B virus
  C. Echovirus
  D. Poliovirus
  E. All enteroviruses

B is correct.
Coxsackie B virus serotypes are associated with neonatal encephalomyocarditis (often acquired during birth) and myocarditis or pericarditis in adults.

251.   Primate cell cultures can be used to isolate all enteroviruses EXCEPT:
  A. Some group B coxsackie virus serotypes
  B. Some group A coxsackie virus serotypes
  C. Some echovirus serotypes
  D. Polioviruses

B is correct.
All enteroviruses can be grown in cell cultures of primate origin except some coxsackie A viruses which require suckling mice for primary isolation. (See also question 181)

252.   The clinical specimen most likely to yield an enteroviral isolate during all phases of illness is:
  A. Throat washings
  B. Blood
  C. Cerebrospinal fluid
  D. Feces
  E. Any of the above

D is correct.
Enteroviruses are shed in the feces during all stages of the disease and for days or weeks after recovery. Throat washings and blood will yield virus only during the early phase and the acute phase, respectively. While coxsackie and echoviruses can be isolated from the CSF during the acute phase, poliovirus does not appear in CSF for reasons not understood.

253.   Regarding host defense mechanisms involved in recovery from enteroviral disease, it can be stated that:
  A. Non-specific defense mechanisms are primarily involved
  B. Cell-mediated responses are solely responsible
  C. Antibody-mediated immunity is solely responsible
  D. Both cell-mediated and antibody-mediated mechanisms are involved, with the antibodies being relatively more important
  E. Both cell-mediated and antibody-mediated mechanisms are involved, with the cell-mediated mechanisms being more important

D is correct.
There is evidence that enteroviral infections are more severe in individuals with defective humoral immunity than in those with defective cell-mediated immunity (CMI). However, CMI is important also because CMI deficiency prolongs the course of enteroviral infections.

254.   Post-polio syndrome (PPS) is described by all of the following statements EXCEPT:
  A. Occurs only in those who have had prior poliomyelitis
  B. The incidence of PPS is higher among women
  C. About 30 years elapse between primary disease and PPS
  D. PPS is characterized by fatigue and pain in muscles affected by primary disease
  E. Poliovirus can be isolated from patients

E is correct.
Poliovirus has not been isolated from PPS patients, and the mechanism whereby prior polio induces PPS years later is not known.

255.   Bulbar poliomyelitis, as opposed to spinal poliomyelitis, is characterized by:
A. Destruction of motor neurons
B. Destruction of spinal neurons
C. Destruction of cranial nerves
D. Paralysis of muscles in limbs
E. All of the above

C is correct.
Bulbar poliomyelitis results from viral destruction of cranial nerves which innervate respiratory muscles. Spinal polio results from killing of spinal neurons which supply muscles in arms and legs. Destruction of motor neurons is common to both types of polio.

256.   All of the following apply to oral poliovirus vaccine (OPV) EXCEPT:
A. A good inducer of cell-mediated immunity
B. Consists of inactivated poliovirus
C. Not recommended to immunize a non-immune adult
D. May not be effective in patients with other enteroviral infections
E. May induce 'herd' immunity

B is correct.
Oral polio vaccine consists of live attenuated poliovirus which may revert to virulence. Hence, it is not recommended for immunizing adults in whom polio is more serious than in children. The virus in OPV is excreted in feces and thereby may immunize non-immune contacts (herd immunity). A current infection with another enterovirus is suspected of interfering with the effectiveness of OPV. In all of the above respects inactivated poliovirus vaccine differs from OPV.

257.   Which of the following statements is true of human rotaviruses?
A. Consist of double-stranded segmented RNA and double-layered capsids
B. They are the major cause of nosocomial diarrhea in the United States
C. They are the primary cause of acute viral diarrhea in children world-wide
D. Enteral immunoglobulin is protective against rotavirus infection
E. All of the above are true

E is correct.

258.   Virus isolated from the feces of a hepatitis patient during the acute phase of the illness consisted of naked virions with single-stranded RNA genome. If this viral isolate were the cause of hepatitis, it could be:
A. Hepatitis A virus (HAV)
B. Hepatitis B virus (HBV) or hepatitis D virus (HDV)
C. Hepatitis C virus (HCV)
D. Hepatitis E virus (HEV)
E. Hepatitis A or E virus (HAV or HEV)

E is correct.
HAV, a picornavirus (enterovirus) and HEV, a calicivirus, both consist of naked virions with single-stranded (+)-sense RNA genomes. HBV (enveloped, partially double-stranded DNA genome) and HCV (enveloped, single-stranded (+)-sense RNA genome) have structural features different from those of HAV or HEV. HDV (delta virus) has the smallest single-stranded RNA genome of any human virus and depends on HBV for its envelope.

259. Hepatitis B virus (HBV) is unique among DNA viruses causing human disease in that:
    A. Its genome is transcribed in the cellular nucleus
    B. Its genome is transcribed by cellular RNA polymerase II
    C. Its virion is enveloped
    D. The replication of its genome involves reverse transcription
    E. It cannot be cultivated *in vitro*

D is correct.
Replication by reverse transcription is the only listed unique feature of hepatitis B virus. The features described by A, B, C and E are true but not unique for HBV. For instance, all DNA viruses except poxviruses are transcribed in the nucleus by cellular RNA polymerase II. (Poxviral genome is transcribed in the cytoplasm by a virus-specific polymerase). Herpesviruses and pox-viruses are also enveloped like HBV. Like HBV, papillomavirus is also a DNA virus which cannot be cultivated *in vitro*.

260. Autonomous replication as well as transmission from patient to patient can be accomplished by all hepatitis viruses EXCEPT:
    A. HBV
    B. HAV
    C. HDV
    D. HCV
    E. HEV

C is correct.
HDV genome, smallest of any human virus, cannot code for coat components involved in attachment to host cells (transmission). It has evolved so as to use HBV envelope as its coat. Without help from HBV, it can direct replication of its genome and cause liver cell injury but cannot spread among hosts.

261. The only hepatitis virus that can be cultivated *in vitro* is:
    A. HAV
    B. HBV
    C. HCV
    D. HDV
    E. HEV

A is correct.
HAV can be grown in primate liver cell cultures. Cultivation *in vitro* has facilitated the production of an inactivated virus vaccine against HAV. None of the other hepatitis viruses can be cultivated *in vitro* as yet.

For questions 262–266, match the numbered epidemiological facts with the lettered hepatitis viruses.
    A. Hepatitis A
    B. Hepatitis B
    C. Hepatitis C
    D. Hepatitis D

262. Transmission is primarily by the oro-fecal route.

A is correct.
The oro-fecal route is the major mode of transmission of HAV (and of HEV).

263. Male gender and early infancy are risk factors for chronic infection with this virus.

B is correct.
Male children less than 2 years old are especially prone to becoming chronically infected with HBV.

264. Infected individuals do not become carriers.

A is correct.
HAV (and HEV) do not cause chronic infection.

265. Most infected persons become carriers.

C is correct.
Almost 75% of HCV-infected persons become carriers as opposed to 10% or less of HBV-infected persons.

266.   Transmitters of this virus also have an active HBV infection.

D is correct.
Without the simultaneous presence of HBV in the patient, HDV cannot obtain its envelope or be transmitted.

For questions 267 and 268, match the lettered markers in blood with the numbered statements concerning hepatitis type B.

   A. HBc antigen
   B. HBs antigen
   C. HBe antigen
   D. Anti-HBs antibody
   E. Anti-HBc antibody

267.   Indicates active viral replication and transmissibility.

C is correct.

268.   Prevents infection with hepatitis B virus.

D is correct.
Hepatitis B virus attaches to host-cell receptors via HBs antigen. Therefore, anti-HBs antigen is protective. HBc and HBe antigens are associated with virion internal components. Antibody against HBc appears early in acute disease well before anti-HBs or anti-HBe, so it is useful in diagnosing acute disease.

For questions 269–272, choose the single best answer.

269.   All of the following are true about hepatitis B EXCEPT:
   A. It has the longest incubation period of all forms of viral hepatitis
   B. It is the most common hepatitis viral infection in the United States
   C. Extrahepatic symptoms occur in hepatitis B patients
   D. It is associated with primary hepatocellular carcinoma
   E. Liver damage in hepatitis B is due to immune mechanisms

B is correct.
The most common hepatitis viral infection in the United States is subclinical infection with hepatitis A virus. All other statements apply to hepatitis B. Extrahepatic symptoms result from immune complex deposition in vessel walls (dermatitis, nephritis) and in joints (arthralgias). Chronic infection with HBV or HBC, is associated with primary hepatocellular carcinoma.

270.   Diagnosis of hepatitis A is usually based on:
   A. Detection of IgM type antibody against HAV in patient's blood
   B. Virus isolation from feces and serological identification
   C. Demonstration of a rise in anti-HAV antibody titer in blood
   D. Detection of HAV-specific antigens in blood
   E. Any of the above procedures

A is correct.
IgM, but not IgG, type antibody indicates recent infection. Virus isolation and demonstration of a rise in antibody titer are both time consuming and unnecessary. HAV-specific antigens do appear in blood in the acute phase of the disease but are not detected routinely for diagnostic purposes.

271. A 25-year-old woman not immune to hepatitis B virus (HBV) learns that she may have been exposed to HBV in the last 24 hours. The best treatment for this patient is administration of:
  A. Hepatitis B immune globulin (HBIG)
  B. HBs antigen vaccine
  C. Immune serum globulin (ISG)
  D. HBIG and HBs antigen vaccine (passive/active immunization)
  E. Any of the above vaccines

D is correct.
Because of the long incubation period for hepatitis B, active immunization with HBs antigen vaccine even after exposure to the virus is protective. However, since the incubation period can be short in some individuals, HBIG is administered first for immediate protection. This is followed by HBs antigen vaccine 24 hours later. Passive/active immunization is the recommended treatment also for a newborn baby congenitally infected with HBV during birth. ISG is used for passive immunization against HAV.

272. The agent that has been successfully used to treat chronic hepatitis B virus infection is:
  A. γ-interferon
  B. α-interferon
  C. HBIG
  D. HBs antigen vaccine
  E. None of the above

B is correct.
α-interferon has been found to be effective in the treatment of chronic hepatitis B and hepatitis C viral infections. HBIG affords only passive, short-lived protection against HBV infection. HBs antigen vaccine is used for active immunization against HBV.

Respiratory Viruses

For questions 273–282, choose the single best answer.

273. All of the following respiratory viruses consist of enveloped virions EXCEPT:
  A. Adenoviruses and rhinoviruses
  B. Paramyxoviruses (measles, mumps, parainfluenza and respiratory syncytial viruses)
  C. Orthomyxoviruses (influenza viruses)
  D. Coronaviruses
  E. Rubella virus

A is correct.
Adenoviruses (double-stranded DNA genome) and rhinoviruses (single-stranded (+)-sense RNA genome) both consist of naked virions.

274. Virions with single-stranded, negative-sense RNA genome and cell entry via fusion of virion envelope with the plasma membrane of the host cell are characteristics of:
  A. Influenza viruses
  B. Coronaviruses
  C. Paramyxoviruses
  D. Rubella virus
  E. All of the above viruses

C is correct.
Paramyxoviruses have negative-sense RNA genomes and enter host cells via fusion. This mode of entry applies only to some enveloped viruses (which include herpesviruses and HIV). Coronaviruses and rubella virus have (+)-sense RNA genomes whereas influenza viruses have (–)-sense, segmented RNA genomes.

275. The emergence of new subtypes of type A influenza virus is attributed to antigenic 'shift'. Which of the following descriptions does NOT apply to antigenic 'shift'?
   A. Probably occurs in a non-human host
   B. Requires coinfection with a human and a non-human type A influenza virus
   C. Involves genome segment reassortment
   D. Produces major changes in the hemagglutinin antigen
   E. Results from mutations in the hemagglutinin gene

E is correct.
All the other statements apply to antigenic shift. Mutations in the hemagglutinin gene produce minor genetic changes known by the term antigenic 'drift'.

276. Functions of the hemagglutinin protein of influenza virus include all of the following EXCEPT:
   A. Promoting release of progeny virions
   B. Attachment to host cells
   C. Induction of protective immunity
   D. Fusion of virion envelope with the membrane of endocytotic vesicles
   E. Agglutination of red blood cells

A is correct.
The neuraminidase glycoprotein on virion surface is believed to play a role in virion release by cleaving cell surface neuraminic (sialic) acid residues to which the progeny virions attach.

277. Which of the following is (are) correct statements about influenza virus-specific mRNA production?
   A. Occurs in the cellular nucleus
   B. Viral genome is transcribed by virus-specific RNA polymerase
   C. Nascent, host mRNA-derived cap structures are used as primers
   D. Inhibition of host mRNA synthesis blocks virus-specific mRNA synthesis as well
   E. All of the above statements are correct

E is correct.
Influenza viruses and retroviruses are the only RNA genome viruses which depend on nuclear functions to produce their mRNAs (influenza virus for mRNA cap structures and retroviruses for transcription of proviral DNA; cellular RNA polymerase activity is essential for both of these requirements).

278. Which of the following is NOT a true statement about the vaccine against influenza virus?
   A. Consists of currently circulating virus strains causing minor epidemics
   B. Consists of inactivated virus
   C. It is not among the most effective viral vaccines
   D. It is recommended mainly for individuals at high risk
   E. Rare complications resulting from vaccination can be effectively treated with amantadine.

E is correct.
Amantadine is protective against type A influenza virus if administered before or within 48 hours after infection. Rare complications from vaccination (e.g. anaphylaxis) occur in individuals allergic to egg protein, traces of which may be present in the vaccine prepared from virus grown in embryonated eggs.

279. All of the following are correct statements about viral influenza EXCEPT:
   A. By weakening mucosal defenses, promotes secondary bacterial infection
   B. Induces transient immunosuppression
   C. Interferon response contributes to clinical symptoms
   D. May cause Reye's syndrome in a rare patient
   E. Viremia is associated with acute illness

E is correct.
Influenza viral infection does not lead to viremia. The mechanism of immunosuppression is unknown. Among typical respiratory viruses viremia is associated with measles and mumps viruses (systemic infection) but not with other paramyxoviruses, coronaviruses or rhinoviruses. Reye's syndrome is associated with aspirin intake by children and teenagers with viral infections, especially type B influenza or chicken pox viral infections.

280. Which of the following is a complication associated with both measles and viral influenza?
   A. Systemic sclerosing panencephalitis (SSPE)
   B. Giant cell pneumonia
   C. Secondary bacterial infections
   D. Pancreatitis
   E. Orchitis

C is correct.
Pneumonia due to secondary bacterial infections is a complication associated with both measles and viral influenza, even though influenza virus may cause pneumonia by itself. Measles virus produces giant cell pneumonia (in children with T-cell deficiency) and the slow viral disease SSPE (in a rare adolescent who has had early childhood measles). Pancreatitis and orchitis are complications associated with mumps.

281. In a patient presenting with respiratory symptoms, high fever and no history of immunization against measles, measles diagnosis can be based on all of the following EXCEPT:
   A. Koplik's spots in the buccal mucosa and syncytia in nasal secretions or urine sediments
   B. Hemagglutination of red blood cells by virus isolated from respiratory secretions
   C. Rash descending from neck to trunk and limbs
   D. Presence of measles virus-specific IgM antibody in patient's blood
   E. Presence of measles virus-specific antigen in clinical specimens

B is correct.
Hemagglutination is a property shared by several respiratory (and other) viruses including measles virus and influenza virus. While specific IgM antibody or antigen will permit definitive diagnosis, in the above patient, Koplik's spots in oral mucosa and syncytia in respiratory secretions as well as descending rash will be highly reliable indicators of measles.

282. To protect a T-cell-deficient child from measles infection, the proper vaccine to be administered is:
   A. Immune serum globulin (ISG)
   B. Killed virus vaccine
   C. Live attenuated virus vaccine
   D. Viral hemagglutinin antigen vaccine
   E. None of the above

A is correct.
Passive immunization via ISG is the only means to protect such a patient who will not be able to mount an immune response to live or inactivated virus or viral antigens. Live attenuated virus in the commonly used vaccine could multiply unchecked in a T-cell-deficient patient with fatal consequences. Inactivated measles virus vaccine is not used even for normal children because (a) it does not protect and (b) it sensitizes the vaccinees to measles viral antigens so that upon subsequent exposure to measles they develop atypical measles. There is no hemagglutinin antigen vaccine against measles.

For questions 283–288, match the numbered statements with the lettered viruses.
   A. Parainfluenza viruses
   B. Mumps virus
   C. Respiratory syncytial virus
   D. All of the above

283. Induces life-long immunity.

B is correct.
Mumps virus produces viremia (like measles virus and rubella virus) and induces long-lasting immunity.

284. Induces short-lived immunity.

A is correct.
Parainfluenza viruses do not produce viremia and produce only short-lived immunity.

285. Induces no immunity and reinfection occurs.

C is correct.
Respiratory syncytial virus, the most important cause of respiratory disease in small infants (bronchiolitis, pneumonia) apparently fails to induce immunity and reinfections occur throughout life.

286. Direct cell-to-cell spread via cell fusion occurs.

D is correct.
All paramyxoviruses have the capacity to spread from infected cells to susceptible cells by inducing fusion between them. The resulting multinucleated cells (syncytia) are a diagnostically useful feature of these infections.

287. Ribavirin is used to treat serious infection.

C is correct.
Ribavirin, a guanosine derivative, is used to treat complications resulting from respiratory syncytial virus infections.

288. Infected cell cultures show positive hemadsorption but no cytopathic effects.

A is correct.
Among paramyxoviruses only parainfluenza viruses fail to produce visible cytopathic effects in cell cultures. However, infected cells express viral hemagglutinin antigen and therefore bind red blood cells (hemadsorption). Thus, hemadsorption aids in laboratory diagnosis of parainfluenza virus infections.

Neurotropic Viruses

For questions 289–297, choose the single best answer.

289. In genome characteristics, mode of replication and virion structure, rabies virus is most closely related to:
    A. California encephalitis virus (CEV)
    B. Herpes simplex virus (HSV)
    C. Eastern equine encephalitis virus (EEV)
    D. Measles virus
    E. St. Louis encephalitis virus (SLEV)

D is correct.
Like measles virus, rabies virus has enveloped virions and a (–)-sense, linear, single-stranded RNA genome. Replication of both viruses involves transcription of subgenome length individual mRNAs and genome length (+)-sense complementary RNA. All of the above viruses are enveloped, but EEV and SLEV genomes are (+)-sense, intact, single-stranded RNA, CEV genome is segmented (–)-sense RNA, and HSV genome is double-stranded DNA.

290.   True statements about rabies include all of the
following EXCEPT:
  A.   There is no human-to-human transmission
  B.   The bite of a rabid animal produces rabies in almost
       all human victims
  C.   Among wild animals sporadic epidemics occur from
       time to time
  D.   Post-exposure prophylaxis includes administration
       of human rabies immunoglobulin and inactivated
       rabies virus vaccine
  E.   With the exception of bats, infected mammals do
       not become carriers

B is correct.
Even though rabies is fatal in almost all victims,
only about 15% of persons bitten by rabid animals
will develop the disease.

291.   Which of the following is NOT a true statement about
rabies?
  A.   The usually long incubation period is shorter if the
       bite wound is in the head
  B.   Viremia is not involved in virus spread to the CNS
  C.   Negribodies can be demonstrated in the cytoplasm
       of infected cells
  D.   Rapid diagnosis is based on immunofluorescent
       detection of viral antigens in the brain cells of
       suspected animals
  E.   Following immunization with the vaccine produced
       in human diploid cell cultures, a few individuals
       develop allergic encephalomyelitis

E is correct.
Allergic encephalomyelitis is a complication
associated with the use of rabbit nerve tissue
vaccine. The current use of virus grown in human
diploid cells has eliminated this problem.

292.   Which of the following virus families contain viruses
that induce meningitis/encephalitis?
  A.   Togaviridae
  B.   Flaviviridae
  C.   Bunyaviridae
  D.   Paramyxoviridae
  E.   All of the above virus families

E is correct.
In addition, some viruses belonging to
Picornaviridae (enteroviruses) and Herpeto-
viridae (herpes simplex virus) are also significant
causes of CNS infection.

293.   Examples of arthropod-borne viruses causing
encephalitis in humans include all of the following
EXCEPT:
  A.   Measles virus
  B.   Eastern equine encephalitis virus
  C.   California encephalitis virus
  D.   Venezuelan encephalitis virus
  E.   St. Louis encephalitis virus

A is correct.
Measles virus often causes encephalitis but is not
an arthropod-borne virus. All other viruses listed
are zoonotic viruses transmitted to humans via
arthropod vectors.

294.   All of the following statements about St. Louis
encephalitis virus are correct EXCEPT:
  A.   It is a flavivirus
  B.   It is related to yellow fever virus and Dengue virus
  C.   It is the most frequent cause of arbovirus
       encephalitis in the United States
  D.   It is transmitted to humans by a tick vector
  E.   It produces mild encephalitis usually without
       neurological sequelae

D is correct.
SLEV is transmitted by mosquitoes. All other
statements apply to SLEV.

295.   True statement(s) about arbovirus cycles in nature include:
   A. Several species serve as hosts for arboviruses
   B. Mosquitoes are susceptible to arboviral disease
   C. Zoonotic hosts serve to amplify arboviral populations
   D. Human-to-human transmission is critical for the survival of most arboviruses
   E. A and C above

E is correct.
Arboviruses infect several species and are amplified in zoonotic hosts. Mosquitoes and other arthropod vectors are persistently infected and do not develop disease. Human-to-human transmission does not occur with most arboviruses (see question 216) and is not critical for their maintenance in nature.

296.   The most frequent cause of acute viral encephalitis in the United States is:
   A. Mumps virus
   B. Measles virus
   C. St. Louis encephalitis virus
   D. Herpes simplex virus
   E. Chicken pox virus

D is correct.
Most adults are latently infected with herpes simplex virus type 1. The latent virus may be reactivated and cause acute encephalitis in an immunocompromised patient.

297.   Examples of viruses which can cause encephalitis long after primary infection include all of the following EXCEPT:
   A. Herpes simplex virus (HSV)
   B. Mumps virus
   C. Rubella virus
   D. Measles virus
   E. The papovavirus JC virus

B is correct.
Encephalitis associated with mumps is a rare complication of acute illness. Acute measles may also involve encephalitis. However, measles, like HSV, rubella virus and JC virus, can persist in the host and become reactivated years later to cause encephalitis. A long interval also elapses between primary HIV infection and AIDS-associated encephalitis.

Herpesviruses

For Questions 298–306, choose the single best answer.

298.   Definitive diagnosis of HSV-encephalitis is based on:
   A. Detection of HSV-specific antigens in temporal lobe biopsy specimen
   B. Elevated leukocyte count in the CSF
   C. Elevated protein content and red cell count in the CSF
   D. Isolation of HSV from CSF
   E. Increased technetium-99 uptake in the temporal lobe

A is correct.
Tissue damage in HSV-encephalitis is localized in the temporal and frontal lobes, and HSV-specific antigens can be readily detected in biopsy specimens. Increased technetium-99 uptake in the temporal lobe is only suggestive evidence, since temporal lobe inflammation due to other causes will also produce this effect. Elevated leukocyte and red cell counts and protein content in the CSF could result from CNS infection by other agents as well. HSV is seldom present in CSF.

299.   All of the following are herpesviruses causing human disease EXCEPT:
   A. B virus of monkeys
   B. Varicella-zoster virus
   C. Marek's disease virus
   D. Herpes simplex virus
   E. Epstein–Barr virus

C is correct.
Marek's disease virus is a herpesvirus causing T-cell lymphomas in chickens. All other viruses listed are herpesviruses causing human disease. B virus of monkeys causes meningoencephalitis in humans. Other herpesviruses causing human disease are cytomegalovirus, human herpes virus-6 (roseola infantum) and the recently discovered Kaposi's sarcoma-associated human herpesvirus.

300. The herpes virus that is a probable cause of certain human cancers is:
   A. Epstein–Barr virus
   B. Cytomegalovirus
   C. Varicella-zoster virus
   D. Herpes simplex virus
   E. Human herpes virus-6

A is correct.
Epstein–Barr virus likely causes Burkitt's lymphoma, B-cell lymphomas in immunodeficient patients, oral hairy leukoplakia in AIDS patients, and nasopharyngeal carcinoma.

301. Which of the following statements apply to all herpes viruses?
   A. All are neurotropic viruses
   B. All of them cause exanthems
   C. All of them cause latent infections
   D. All of them transform cells *in vitro*
   E. All of the above

C is correct.
Reactivation of latent herpesviruses in immunocompromised patients is a major medical problem. Neurotropism is primarily associated with herpes simplex virus, chicken pox virus, and the B virus of monkeys. Cytomegalovirus causes CNS disease in AIDS patients. Other herpesviruses are not neurotropic. Exanthems are produced by herpes simplex virus, chicken pox virus and human herpes simplex virus-6 (roseola infantum) but not by the other herpesviruses. Chicken pox virus does not transform cells.

302. The human herpesvirus that is often acquired via transfusions and transplantations is:
   A. Cytomegalovirus (CMV)
   B. Herpes simplex virus (HSV)
   C. Epstein–Barr virus (EBV)
   D. Varicella-zoster virus (VZV)
   E. None of the above

A is correct.
CMV remains latent in leukocytes and is often transmitted via transplanted organs (e.g. kidney) or blood transfusions. EBV may be acquired through blood transfusions, but seldom through transplants. HSV and VZV are not transmitted by these means.

303. Socioeconomic factors are NOT important determinants of infections caused by:
   A. Cytomegalovirus
   B. Varicella-zoster virus (VZV)
   C. Epstein–Barr virus
   D. Herpes simplex virus
   E. Any of the above viruses

B is correct.
The incidence of infection with respiratory viruses such as VZV is the same among all children regardless of their socioeconomic status. Saliva contact is the major mode of transmission of the other herpesviruses mentioned. Infections by viruses transmitted via saliva contact or ingestion are more prevalent among children living under poor living conditions.

304. Some herpesviruses are transmitted by more than one mechanism. Multiple modes of transmission apply best to:
   A. Epstein–Barr virus (EBV)
   B. Herpes simplex virus (HSV)
   C. Varicella-zoster virus (VZV)
   D. Cytomegalovirus (CMV)
   E. All of the above viruses equally

D is correct.
CMV is transmitted transplacentally, sexually, and through breast milk, saliva contact, kidney transplants and transfusions.

305. A newborn baby shows symptoms of cytomegalic inclusion disease and a high blood titer of IgM type antibody against CMV. The baby is likely to have acquired this infection:
- A. *In utero*, due to reactivation of maternal latent infection
- B. During birth from cervical secretions
- C. Soon after birth, from the mother, via breast milk
- D. *In utero*, from the mother, who acquired primary CMV infection during pregnancy
- E. By none of the above means

D is correct.
This disease in newborn babies results from intrauterine infection with CMV. If the mother had a latent infection at the time of pregnancy, she will have antibody capable of protecting the fetus. It is more likely that the non-immune mother became infected in pregnancy and, in turn, infected the fetus before producing IgG type anti-CMV antibodies. CMV infection of the baby during or after birth usually does not cause disease.

306. In a young adult lymphocytosis with morphologically atypical lymphocytes could be the result of infection with:
- A. Cytomegalovirus
- B. Herpes simplex virus
- C. Varicella-zoster virus
- D. Epstein–Barr virus
- E. A or D above

E is correct.
The blood picture described is typical of mononucleosis which could be caused by EBV, or on rare occasion by CMV in non-immune young adults. EBV-mononucleosis (infectious mononucleosis) but not CMV-mononucleosis is often associated with a heterophile antibody in the blood. The presence of this antibody in patient blood can be demonstrated by the mononucleosis spot test.

For questions 307 and 308, match the lettered viruses with the numbered statements.
- A. Cytomegalovirus (CMV)
- B. Epstein–Barr virus (EBV)
- C. Herpes simplex virus (HSV)
- D. Varicella-zoster virus (VZV)

307. Requires B lymphocytes for *in vitro* growth.

B is correct.
EBV preferentially infects B cells even though it infects epithelial cells also. EBV enters B cells via attachment to the complement (C3d) receptor CR2 on B-cell surface.

308. Grows in cell cultures derived from different species.

C is correct.
HSV grows in cell cultures of diverse origin and is therefore relatively easy to isolate. CMV requires primary human fibroblast cell cultures for growth *in vitro*. VZV can be cultivated in primary or continuous human-derived cell cultures.

For questions 309–313, choose the single best answer.

309. Complications resulting from chicken pox include all of the following EXCEPT:
- A. Shingles
- B. Fetal infection
- C. Encephalitis
- D. Pneumonia
- E. Reye's syndrome

A is correct.
Shingles is not a complication of chicken pox but the result of latent chicken pox virus (in dorsal ganglia) becoming reactivated at a later time in immunocompromised patients. In pregnant mothers with chicken pox, the fetal infection rate is about 2%. Regarding Reye's syndrome, see question 279. Complications are more likely to occur in adults and immunocompromised patients.

310.   All of the following are correct statements about Epstein–Barr virus (EBV) latency EXCEPT:
   A.   Latently infected host cells are B lymphocytes
   B.   Latently infected cells grow in culture indefinitely (immortalization)
   C.   Viral genome replicates in latently infected cells without virion production
   D.   Host cell DNA polymerase replicates viral genome in latently infected cells
   E.   Latently infected cells may give rise to lymphomas in immunodeficient patients

D is correct.
All herpesviruses, including EBV virus, code for their own DNA polymerase, but use cellular RNA polymerase II to transcribe their genomes. EBV DNA polymerase is one of the few proteins expressed in latently infected B-lymphocytes.

311.   Which of the following statements is NOT true about herpes simplex virus infections?
   A.   During infection with HSV-1 or HSV-2, the antibody response is type-specific
   B.   The sera of latently infected individuals will contain anti-HSV antibodies
   C.   Both types of HSV can spread directly from cell to cell and thereby escape detection by antibodies
   D.   HSV-specific antigens appearing on infected cell surface permit rapid diagnosis by immuno-fluorescence
   E.   Eosinophilic nuclear inclusion bodies produced in infected cells are diagnostically useful

A is correct.
Not only type-specific antibodies but also cross-reacting antibodies will be induced by either serotype since they share many antigens.

312.   All of the following antiviral agents used to treat herpesviral diseases are nucleoside analogs EXCEPT:
   A.   Ara-A
   B.   Ganciclovir
   C.   Acyclovir
   D.   Foscarnet
   E.   IUdR

D is correct.
Foscarnet (trisodium phosphonoformate) is a pyrophosphate analog and is active as it is. The other agents are all nucleoside analogs and have to be phosphorylated to become antivirally active nucleotide analogs. Foscarnet is useful to treat ganciclovir-resistant CMV infections and acyclovir-resistant HSV infections.

313.   Correct statements about acyclovir include all of the following EXCEPT:
   A.   It is converted into the antivirally active form in HSV-infected cells but not in uninfected cells
   B.   It is relatively nontoxic
   C.   It inhibits HSV-specific thymidine kinase (HSV-TK)
   D.   It blocks HSV-specific DNA synthesis
   E.   It is especially effective in preventing HSV disease in immunocompromised patients

C is correct.
HSV-TK is not inhibited by acyclovir (Acyclo G). In fact, HSV-TK phosphorylates Acyclo G producing the mononucleotide (Acyclo GMP). A cellular kinase then converts Acyclo GMP into the antivirally active trinucleotide (Acyclo GTP). Acyclo GTP inhibits HSV-specific DNA polymerase much more than it inhibits host cell DNA polymerase. Normal cellular TK does not phosphorylate acyclovir. Thus, acyclovir is targeted to HSV-infected cells and HSV-specific DNA synthesis.

For questions 314–316, match the herpesviral diseases with the antiherpetic agents used to treat them.

    A. Ara-A
    B. Acyclovir
    C. Ganciclovir
    D. IUdR
    E. None of the above

314. CMV-induced pneumonia in AIDS patients.

C is correct.
Ara-A, IUdR and acyclovir are ineffective against CMV.

315. Pneumonia associated with chicken pox complications.

B is correct.
Acyclovir, but none of the others, may be useful to treat complications resulting from chicken pox.

316. Mononucleosis caused by Epstein–Barr virus (EBV).

E is correct.
None of the available antiherpetic agents is useful to treat EBV-infections.

Retroviruses

For questions 317–323, choose the single best answer.

317. Structural features of human immune deficiency virus (HIV) include all of the following EXCEPT:
    A. Enveloped virions
    B. Cylindrical virion core
    C. Bullet-shaped virions
    D. Diploid RNA genome
    E. Reverse transcriptase in virions

C is correct.
HIV virions are spherical. Bullet-shaped virions are characteristic of rabies virus and other rhabdoviruses.

318. Which of the following statements is NOT true about the tat protein of HIV?
    A. It is a virion structural component
    B. It has been shown to induce apoptosis in T lymphocytes
    C. It enhances HIV genome transcription
    D. It is essential for HIV replication
    E. All of the above statements are true

A is correct.
Tat is a regulatory protein specified by HIV but not found in the virion structure. Rev is the other essential regulatory protein which increases HIV-specific message in the cell.

319. Correct statements about the epidemiology of HIV-infection include all of the following EXCEPT:
    A. HIV-type 1 and HIV-type 2 are equally pathogenic
    B. HIV-1 subtype E may be more adept at heterosexual transmission than subtype B
    C. Infected seropositive individuals are carriers of HIV
    D. HIV is vertically transmitted from mother to baby
    E. Men and women are equally susceptible to HIV-infection

A is correct.
HIV-2 is far less pathogenic than HIV-1 and requires 25 years or so to produce immune deficiency in the host.

320. The body fluid through which HIV is NOT known to be transmitted is:
    A. Semen
    B. Saliva
    C. Blood
    D. Breast milk

B is correct.
HIV transmission through saliva contact has not been documented.

321. All of the following are true statements about HIV–host cell interaction EXCEPT:
    A. HIV receptor on host T cells is involved in antigen recognition by these cells
    B. HIV attaches to host cells via the virion surface molecule gp^{41}
    C. Cells in which HIV replicates can fuse with susceptible cells to form syncytia
    D. HIV replicates in macrophages for prolonged periods
    E. HIV-infection of helper T cells may be productive or latent

B is correct.
HIV virions attach to CD4 molecules on host cells via gp^{120}. gp^{41} is the transmembrane protein which induces fusion between HIV envelope and the plasma membrane or HIV-infected cells and susceptible cells. Syncytium formation is a diagnostically useful characteristic. Productive infection occurs in activated (proliferating) T helper cells and latent infection in resting T helper cells.

322. Which of the following statements about anti-HIV antibodies is (are) correct?
    A. Anti-HIV antibodies appear within weeks after infection
    B. HIV can spread from cell to cell without coming into contact with antibodies
    C. Some anti-HIV antibodies may enhance HIV infection
    D. Diagnosis of HIV infection can be based on detection of anti-HIV antibodies in blood
    E. All of the above

E is correct.
All answers including C are correct. Antibody-coated HIV particles are readily taken up by macrophages in which HIV can multiply. Therefore, anti-HIV antibodies may facilitate rather than prevent HIV infection.

323. Which of the following is true of the patient with full-blown AIDS?
    A. Only a low level of plasma viremia can be detected
    B. $CD4^+$ cell count is still high, but begins to decline slowly
    C. The lymph nodes are more or less intact functionally and structurally
    D. The immune response is drastically compromised
    E. Lymphadenopathy is a characteristic symptom

D is correct.
In a patient with full-blown AIDS, severe depletion of $CD4^+$ cell number and destruction of lymphoid organs have already taken place, hence the loss of immune function resulting in opportunistic infections. High levels of viremia are typical of this stage. Low levels of viremia, with slow decline in $CD4^+$ cell count and more or less intact lymph nodes are typical of the long asymptomatic phase of the disease which precedes full-blown AIDS. Lymphadenopathy, transient high level of plasma viremia, and a vigorous immune response are characteristic of the first stage (acute phase) of infection which lasts for 10–12 weeks.

For questions 324–328, match the lettered answers with the numbered statements.

    A. Protease inhibitors
    B. Reverse transcriptase inhibitors
    C. Both of the above
    D. Neither of the above

324.   Give rise to drug-resistant mutants of HIV.

C is correct.
Drug-resistant viral mutants arise during treatment with both classes of agents. Early initiation of treatment with a regimen combining reverse transcriptase inhibitors and a protease inhibitor minimizes the emergence of drug resistance.

325.   Target a host cell-specific enzyme involved in HIV replication.

D is correct.
The targets of these agents are HIV-specific protease and reverse transcriptase.

326.   Arrest ongoing virion production in HIV-infected cells.

D is correct.
Neither class of agents can arrest ongoing virion production because in virus-producing cells, reverse transcription and integration of viral genetic information into host genome have already taken place and protease inhibitors do not block virion production (see question 327 below).

327.   Allows production of non-infectious virions in HIV-infected cells.

A is correct.
Protease inhibitors prevent processing of the precursors of HIV-specific proteins. As a result, virions containing unprocessed envelope glycoproteins are produced. Such virions are non-infectious.

328.   Protects cells from productive HIV infection.

C is correct.
Both types of agents prevent infection of new host cells because virions produced in the presence of protease inhibitors are non-infectious and reverse transcriptase inhibitors prevent proviral DNA synthesis, an essential early event in retrovirus replication.

For questions 329–334, choose the single best answer.

329.   Acute leukemia viruses of other species:
    A. Are replication defective
    B. Readily transform host cells *in vitro*
    C. Carry in their genomes a host cell derived oncogene
    D. Are not transmitted vertically
    E. Are described by all of the above

E is correct.
All of the above are definitive characteristics of acute leukemia viruses of other mammals and birds. Human T-cell leukemia virus, which causes acute leukemia in humans, is not replication defective and does not contain a host-derived oncogene in its genome. (See question 332 below.)

330.   Which of the following attributes applies to DNA tumor viruses but NOT to RNA tumor viruses?
  A. Either transform or replicate in host cells but do not do both
  B. Replication does not result in cell-killing, but may cause cell transformation
  C. May contain in their genomes a host-derived oncogene
  D. Transformation requires viral genome replication and gene expression
  E. None of the above

331.   Correct statements concerning the epidemiology of human T-cell leukemia virus (HTLV-1) include all of the following EXCEPT:
  A. HTLV-1 causes rapidly fatal acute leukemia
  B. Infection with HTLV-1 is rare but equally prevalent in all populations
  C. In the United States, intravenous drug users are at high risk for HTLV-1 infection
  D. HTLV-1 infection has an incubation period of several years
  E. There is evidence for sexual and placental transmission of HTLV-1

332.   Concerning tumor induction by HTLV-1, all of the following statements are correct EXCEPT:
  A. Host cells are helper T lymphocytes
  B. Transforms primate T lymphocytes *in vitro*
  C. Contains a human-derived oncogene in its genome
  D. Codes for a protein which induces expression of growth-promoting host cell proteins
  E. Tumor cells contain HTLV-1-specific sequences

333.   Which of the following statements concerning human papillomaviruses (HPV) is NOT true?
  A. HPV-specific DNA can be detected in the vast majority of cases of cervical intraepithelial neoplasia
  B. The serotypes most frequently associated with cervical cancer are HPV-16, and to a lesser extent HPV-18
  C. The early gene products E6 and E7 proteins of these viruses inactivate tumor suppressor proteins
  D. Papillomaviruses can be readily isolated by growth in cell cultures
  E. HPV-16 and HPV-18 are transmitted sexually

A is correct.
DNA tumor viruses transform only those host cells in which they cannot replicate. Permissive host cells in which they replicate are killed. Statements B, C and D apply to RNA tumor viruses. DNA tumor viruses code for one or more early expressed proteins which alone, in the absence of viral genome replication, can cause cell transformation. These proteins promote cell proliferation by binding to and inactivating tumor suppressor proteins such as p53.

B is correct.
There are endemic areas such as Southwest Japan where the infection rate is higher than in the rest of the world. All other statements apply to HTLV-1.

C is correct.
HTLV-1 is unique among acute leukemia-sarcoma viruses in that its genome does not contain a host-derived oncogene. HTLV-1 codes for a protein which through transactivation induces the expression of growth-promoting host cell molecules such as IL-2, IL-2 receptor and the oncoprotein c-fos, and thereby, presumably, causes cell transformation.

D is correct.
Papillomaviruses will not grow in cell cultures. They infect and transform basal epithelial cells (squamous cells) without producing progeny. Progeny virions are produced only as the squamous cells differentiate into keratinocytes. Keratinocytes will not grow in culture. Diagnosis is by detection of virus-specific DNA following amplification by PCR.

334.   Epstein–Barr virus (EBV) is implicated in which of the following human tumors?
    A. Oral hairy leukoplakia (OHL)
    B. Burkitt's lymphoma (BL)
    C. Polyclonal lymphoma
    D. Nasopharyngeal carcinoma
    E. All of the above

E is correct.

OHL is the name for papillomatous lesions along the edge of the tongue resulting from EBV-induced epithelial cell proliferation in AIDS patients. BL is endemic in Central Africa and New Guinea and associated with EBV-induced c-myc oncogene expression in B lymphocytes. Where BL is endemic, an additional factor in the development of BL is believed to be malarial parasite-induced immunosuppression allowing EBV-transformed B cells to proliferate.

V.   MICROBIOLOGY

General Microbiology

For questions 335–337, match the lettered type of microscopy with the appropriate numbered statement.

   A. Darkfield microscopy
   B. Phase-contrast microscopy
   C. Compound light microscopy
   D. Fluorescence microscopy

335.   The type of microscopy most often used for observing stained bacterial smears.

C is correct.
Also known as brightfield microscopy, compound light microscopy using an oil immersion lens to reduce light loss is used for observing most stained specimens.

336.   Uses an ultraviolet or near-ultraviolet source of illumination and is commonly employed in diagnostic procedures.

D is correct.
Fluorescence microscopy with or without specific antibody and with fluorochrome dyes is used to observe bacteria such as *Treponema pallidum* and *Mycobacterium tuberculosis*.

337.   The most useful microscopy for observing the presence of very small, unstained organisms.

A is correct.
Darkfield microscopy makes a light silhouette of the object against a black background. Certain organisms such as spirochetes are readily visible.

For questions 338–340, match the lettered type of stain with the appropriate lettered statement.

   A. Gram-positive
   B. Gram-negative
   C. Acid-fast
   D. All of the above

338.   The crystal violet-iodine complex is retained by a thick layer of peptidoglycan in the cell wall.

A is correct.
Gram-positive bacteria are not decolorized by alcohol washing because the peptidoglycan layer in the cell wall traps crystal violet–iodine complex.

339.   Counterstained material appears blue.

C is correct.
The acid-fast stain uses methylene blue to stain all non-acid-fast material.

340.   Alcohol washing disrupts the lipopolysaccharide outer membrane of these bacteria.

B is correct.
Gram-negative bacteria become colorless after alcohol washing because the peptidoglycan layer in their cell wall is very thin, and the lipids in their outer membrane are soluble.

For questions 341–344, match the lettered kingdom with the appropriate numbered statement.

A. Eukaryotes
B. Prokaryotes
C. Both of the above
D. Neither of the above

341. Their cytoplasmic membranes contain sterol.

A is correct.
Only eurkaryotes contain sterols in their membranes. The exceptions are the prokaryotes that belong to the genera *Mycoplasma* and *Ureaplasma*.

342. Respiration is via cytoplasmic membrane.

B is correct.
Respiration is associated with the cytoplasmic membranes in prokaryotes and with mitochondria in eurkaryotes.

343. The genome or genetic material may be either RNA or DNA.

D is correct.
The genomes of both prokaryotes and eurkaryotes are in the form of DNA. Only viruses may have either DNA or RNA as genetic material.

344. The cell wall, if present, contains peptidoglycan.

B is correct.
Peptidoglycan is unique to bacteria. The cell walls of eukaryotes are composed of cellulose or chitin.

For questions 345–352, choose the single best answer.

345. Which of the following is NOT associated with the peptidoglycan layer of bacterial cell walls?
    A. Rigidity and cell shape
    B. Target for β-lactam antibiotics
    C. Fever induction (pyrogenic activity)
    D. Irreversible shock and cardiovascular collapse

D is correct.
Although sometimes associated with chronic inflammatory responses, peptidoglycan is not responsible for shock and cardiovascular collapse observed in some gram-negative infections.

346. Which of the following functions is associated with bacterial capsule?
    A. Provide specific adherence
    B. Serve as an antiphagocytic surface
    C. Protect from environmental hazards
    D. All of the above

D is correct.
In certain species of bacteria the capsule can function in all of the above capacities.

347. Which combination of cell wall components consists of unique elements of gram-negative and gram-positive bacterial cell walls and serves as a virulence factor?
    A. Lipopolysaccharide-teichoic acid
    B. Peptidoglycan-core polysaccharide
    C. Phospholipid-pore proteins
    D. Teichoic acid-peptidoglycan

A is correct.
Lipopolysaccharide (LPS) is the endotoxin component of gram-negative bacteria. Teichoic acid is a component unique to gram-positive bacteria that serves to attach the cells to specific receptors on mammalian cells.

348. When flagella proteins are used for serological classification, they are referred to as:
   A. O-antigen
   B. H-antigen
   C. K-antigen
   D. Vi-antigen

B is correct.
The H-antigen is flagellar protein. The O-antigen is the outer polysaccharide surface antigen frequently used in laboratory diagnosis of gram-negative bacteria. K-antigens are the polysaccharide components of encapsulated organisms such as *Klebsiella* and certain strains of *E. coli*. The Vi-antigens are capsular virulence antigens used for typing of *Salmonella typhi*.

349. Which of the following statements is NOT true regarding bacterial spores?
   A. They are an alternative means of reproduction for members of the genera *Bacillus* and *Clostridium*
   B. The process of sporulation includes the synthesis of dipicolinic acid
   C. Spore formation is accompanied by the uptake of calcium and dehydration
   D. Germination can be stimulated either by mild heat or presence of certain amino acids

A is correct.
A spore is formed from a single vegetative cell and germinates to yield a new vegetative cell. Thus, it is not a means of reproduction but rather a resistant dormant body.

350. The primary function of fimbriae is to:
   A. Promote transfer of DNA between bacterial cells
   B. Provide an antiphagocytic surface
   C. Mediate specific adherence of bacteria to other bacteria and mammalian cells
   D. Serve as receptors for specific IgA immunoglobulins

C is correct.
Fimbriae mediate the adherence of bacteria to cells and are particularly important in the colonization of mucosal surfaces.

351. The presence of pili on the surface of a bacterial cell indicates that the cell:
   A. Can serve as a donor of DNA
   B. Is gram-negative
   C. May possess a large plasmid
   D. All of the above

D is correct.
Pili are structures used for transfer of DNA, including plasmids by some gram-negative bacteria.

352. The purified form of endotoxin found in the outer membrane of gram-negative bacteria is:
   A. O-antigen
   B. Lipid-A
   C. Peptidoglycan
   D. Teichoic acid

B is correct.
Purified lipid-A can mimic the effects of endotoxin.

Morphology

For questions 353 and 354, match the appropriate lettered structure in the figure below with the appropriate numbered statement.

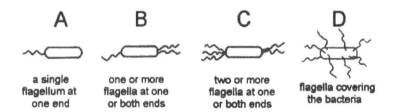

A	B	C	D
a single flagellum at one end	one or more flagella at one or both ends	two or more flagella at one or both ends	flagella covering the bacteria

353. The term used to describe that arrangement of flagella depicted in figure C is:
   A. Monotrichous
   B. Amphitrichous
   C. Lophotrichous
   D. Peritrichous

D is correct.
Peritrichous describes the random arrangement of flagella scattered around the bacterial cell.

354. The arrangement of the flagellum observed in figure A is similar to that seen in motile species of:
   A. *Proteus*
   B. *Escherichia*
   C. *Pseudomonas*
   D. *Salmonella*

C is correct.
Pseudomonas species possess a single, polar (monotrichous) flagellum.

For questions 355–358, match the appearance of the lettered shape in the figure below with that of the organism that causes the numbered disease.

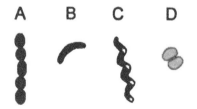

A   B   C   D

355.   Cholera.

B is correct.
Vibrio cholerae, a slightly curved gram-negative rod.

356.   Syphilis.

C is correct.
Treponema pallidum, a flexible, helical shape.

357.   Scarlet fever.

A is correct.
Streptococcus pyogenes divides in one plane, and the daughters remains attached in chain-like patterns.

358.   Pneumococcal pneumonia.

D is correct.
Streptococcus pneumoniae divides in one plane and remains attached as diplococcus.

Growth Characteristics

For questions 359 and 360, match the lettered term for the preferred growth temperature with the appropriate numbered statement.

A. Mesophiles
B. Thermophiles
C. Psychrophiles
D. Hyperthermophiles

359. The term used to describe the preferred temperature range of most pathogenic bacteria.

A is correct.
Mesophiles or moderate temperature-loving microbes.

360. The group of microbes most commonly responsible for food spoilage.

C is correct.
Refrigeration is the most common method of food preservation, therefore organisms that grow at temperatures of 0–30°C cause most food spoilage.

For questions 361–364, match the lettered term for oxygen requirements with the appropriate numbered statement.

A. Obligate aerobes
B. Facultative anaerobes
C. Obligate anaerobes
D. Microaerophilic

361. The causative agent of tuberculosis.

A is correct.
Mycobacterium tuberculosis is an obligate aerobe which frequently produces lesions in the lung apex where there is high oxygen tension.

362. The cause of traveler's diarrhea.

B is correct.
Enterotoxigenic *E. coli*, a facultative anaerobe.

363. This bacterium is capable of both aerobic and anaerobic growth, but it grows better in the presence of oxygen.

B is correct.
A facultative anaerobe. In these organisms, both superoxide dismutase (converts superoxide to H_2O_2) and catalase (breaks down H_2O_2 to H_2O and O_2) enzymes are present, and hydrogen atoms are combined with oxygen to form water. Since respiration yields more energy than fermentation, growth is better in the presence of oxygen.

364. Oxygen is required in low concentrations.

D is correct.
Microaerophilic organisms. Bacteria such as *Campylobacter jejuni* require a reduced oxygen atmosphere (about 5%) to grow optimally. They survive only in niches with reduced oxygen.

For questions 365 and 366, match the lettered phases of bacterial growth in the figure below with the appropriate numbered statement.

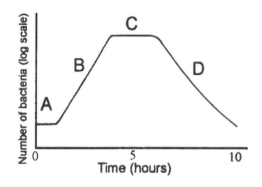

365. In which phase of growth does the cell population show no net increase due to low metabolic activity caused by the exhaustion of nutrients or harmful changes in the environment?

C is correct.
The stationary phase. This phase is a period of equilibrium where the number of microbial deaths balances the number of new cells produced by cell divisions.

366. During which phase are the micro-organisms particularly sensitive to adverse conditions?

B is correct.
During the logarithmic phase, micro-organisms are most active metabolically and are most susceptible to radiation, antimicrobial drugs, etc.

Antimicrobial Agents

For questions 367– 370, match the basic structures lettered A–D in the figure below with the appropriate class of numbered antimicrobial agents.

367. Tetracyclines.

A is correct.
A broad spectrum antibiotic with bacteriostatic activity. A reversible inhibitor of protein synthesis.

368. Chloramphenicol.

C is correct.
A broad spectrum antibiotic with bacteriostatic activity. An inhibitor of protein synthesis with good permeability across the blood–brain barrier.

369. Penicillins.

B is correct.
All penicillins are derivatives of this 6-amino-penicillanic acid. The basic structure is a β-lactam ring linked to a thiazolidine ring.

370. Fluoroquinolones.

D is correct.
These broad spectrum bactericidal antibiotics are related to nalidixic acid and act by inhibiting DNA gyrase.

For questions 371–373, match the BEST lettered germicides with the numbered application.

A. Silver nitrate and/or silver sulfadiazine
B. 0.5% iodine + 70% alcohol
C. Ethylene oxide
D. 2% aqueous glutaraldehyde
E. 0.5–3% phenolic aqueous solutions

371. Skin antiseptic.

B is correct.

372. Antiseptics especially for ophthalmology and burn patients.

A is correct.

373. Sterilization of biologicals and equipment that would be damaged by heat.

C is correct.

For questions 374–379, match the lettered mechanism of resistance with the appropriate numbered antibiotic and bacteria.

A. Failure to enter the cell (intrinsic resistance)
B. Alteration in membrane proteins (decreased uptake)
C. Alterations in membrane transport systems (efflux)
D. Enzymatic inactivation of antibiotic
E. Alteration in RNA polymerase
F. Alterations in ribosomal proteins
G. Methylation of 23S RNA
H. Altered DNA gyrase
I. More than one of the above

374. Quinolones (nalidixic acid, etc.) – *Enterobacteriaceae*.

H is correct.
Nalidixic acid and related quinolones inhibit the A subunit of DNA gyrase.

375. β-lactams – *Pseudomonas* sp.

I is correct.
The β-lactam antibiotics may be ineffective against *Pseudomonas* sp. because of its failure to enter the cell or by enzymatic inactivation of the drug by β-lactamase.

376. Tetracyclines – *Streptococcus, Enterobacteriaceae*.

C is correct.
New membrane transport systems prevent the tetracyclines from entering the cell.

377.   Chloramphenicol – *S. aureus, Enterobacteriaceae.*

I is correct.
Resistance to chloramphenicol may develop by enzymatic inactivation, by chloramphenicol acetyltransferase, or by impaired transport of the drug into the cell after enzymatic alterations.

378.   Streptomycin – *Enterobacteriaceae.*

F is correct.
Alteration of the S12 protein of the 30S ribosome alters the target of this antibiotic.

379.   Erythromycin – *S. aureus, Streptococcus epidermidis, Enterobacteriaceae.*

I is correct.
Resistance to erythromycin can develop by either the methylation of the 23S RNA as in the case of *S. aureus* or by active efflux by a new membrane transport system by *Enterobacteriaceae* and *Streptococcus epidermidis.*

For question 380, use the lettered precipitation pattern in the figure below.

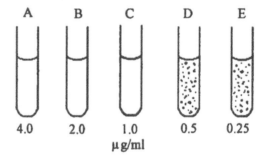

380.   Based on the bacterial growth pattern of the dilution susceptibility test depicted above, the MIC for this organism is:
    A. 4.0 μg/ml
    B. 2.0 μg/ml
    C. 1.0 μg/ml
    D. 0.5 μg/ml
    E. 0.25 μg/ml

C is correct.
The least amount of antimicrobic required to prevent any visible growth is the minimum inhibitory concentration (MIC) for the organism.

Bacterial Genetics

For questions 381–385, match the numbered statement with the lettered type of genetic change.

    A. Bacterial transformation
    B. Generalized transduction
    C. Specialized transduction
    D. Conjugation

381.   The mode of transfer of the DNA is by passive diffusion through the medium.

A is correct.
The transforming DNA is liberated into the medium following the lysis of donor cells.

382.   Which mechanism of gene transfer can be mediated only by a temperate bacteriophage following the lysogenic pathway?

C is correct.
Specialized transduction requires the improper excision of a prophage from the bacterial chromosome which can be accomplished only by a temperate phage in a lysogenized cell.

383.   Newly acquired genetic material is integrated into the bacterial chromosome by site-specific recombination.

C is correct.
During specialized transduction the prophage carrying a bacterial gene recombines with the bacterial chromosome only at a site containing specific base sequences.

384.   Which method of genetic exchange has the potential for transferring the largest number of genetic traits in a single event?

D is correct.
Conjugation can involve the mobilization and transfer of the bacterial chromosome in Hfr donor cells.

385.   This method involves the transfer of a single strand of DNA though a pilus.

D is correct.
Conjugation results in the transfer of a single strand of either plasmid or chromosomal DNA through a pilus.

For questions 386 and 387, match the numbered statement with the appropriate lettered type of transduction.

   A. Specialized transduction
   B. Generalized transduction
   C. Both of the above
   D. Neither of the above

386.   Transducing particles arise during the lytic growth of a bacteriophage.

B is correct.
Generalized transduction results from the packaging of bacterial DNA into phage heads during lytic phage growth.

387.   Inheritance of the transduced traits requires two DNA cross-overs mediated by the bacteria's *rec* genes (recombination genes).

B is correct.
Generalized transduction occurs when there is a replacement of homologous recipient DNA by the transducing DNA. Homologous recombination will then occur with bacterial recombination-repair enzymes.

For questions 388–390, match the numbered statement with the appropriate lettered heading.

   A. Transformation in *Haemophilus influenzae*
   B. Transformation in *Streptococcus pneumoniae*
   C. Both of the above
   D. Neither of the above

388.   Requires the presence of an external competence factor.

B is correct.
External competence factors induce intracellular events that allow *S. pneumoniae* to bind and take up exogenous DNA for transformation.

389. Only closely-related homologous DNA can be bound and taken up into the cell.

A is correct.
Only DNA with specific base sequences can bind and be taken up by *H. influenzae* cells.

390. The transforming DNA is incorporated into the bacterial chromosome as a single strand.

C is correct.
A single strand of transforming DNA displaces one of the native DNA strands in the transforming cell. Following DNA replication, one daughter cell exhibits the original phenotype and the other daughter cell has a newly inherited trait.

For questions 391 and 392, match the numbered statement with the appropriate lettered heading.

A. Deletion mutation
B. Repressor protein
C. Phenotypic lag
D. Suppressor mutation

391. A mutation that can change the effects of another mutation.

D is correct.
An example is an alteration in a transfer RNA anticodon so that it would recognize one of the termination codons as an amino acid codon and thus suppress a nonsense mutation.

392. A genetic alteration that cannot revert back to the wildtype phenotype.

A is correct.
A deletion mutant results from loss of one or more bases and thus cannot revert back to the original state.

In vitro amplification of nucleic acids has been developed for the rapid identification of infectious agents as well as their genes for toxin production and resistance.

For questions 393–397, match the lettered amplification method with the numbered enzyme(s) used to carry out these reactions.

A. Polymerase chain reaction (PCR)
B. Strand displacement amplification (SDA)
C. Transcription-based amplification (TAS or 3SR)
D. DNA ligase-dependent amplification (LCR)
E. bDNA-based signal amplifications

393. Thermophilic DNA polymerase.

A is correct.
PCR utilizes DNA polymerase for the synthesis of complementary strands from heat denatured DNA. Thermophilic DNA polymerase is resistant to denaturation during the heating cycles which allows the amplification to continue.

394. Thermophilic DNA ligase.

D is correct.
The LCR reaction joins mixed primers after they have annealed to denatured target sequences. Thermophilic ligase is resistant to the heating which denatures the target DNA and allows the cycle to continue.

395. Reverse transcriptase and RNA polymerase.

C is correct.

Transcription-based amplification systems make a DNA copy from RNA target molecules. Some techniques (3SR) also use RNase H to remove RNA from RNA–DNA hybrid molecules and convert the molecules to cDNA.

396. This amplification method does NOT employ the use of enzymes.

E is correct.

bDNA hybridizes to extender probes which in turn provide multiple signals for hybridization with labeled probes. The hybridization is based on complementary bases and does not require enzymatic reactions.

397. Restriction endonucleases and DNA polymerase.

B is correct.

SDA technology is based on the ability to generate site-specific nicks by restriction endonuclease. DNA polymerase then initiates DNA synthesis at the single-stranded nick which is within a target DNA.

For questions 398–401, choose the single best answer.

398. The transfer of the F factor during conjugation:
    A. Requires the replication of the F plasmid
    B. Converts the recipient to an F+ donor cell
    C. Requires a pilus encoded by the F+ plasmid
    D. Does not change the phenotype of the donor cell
    E. All of the above

E is correct.

399. Which of the following characteristics is NOT true regarding LARGE plasmids?
    A. They replicate under relaxed control which produces many copies per cell
    B. They usually change the phenotype of the host cell
    C. They show plasmid incompatibility for closely-related plasmids
    D. They may be conjugative and initiate their transfer to other cells
    E. They use DNA polymerase III for their replication

A is correct.

The replication of large plasmids is well regulated and their copy numbers per cell are low.

400. Bacterial chromosomal genes are NOT transferred from one cell to another during:
    A. Restricted (specialized) transduction
    B. Conjugation between F+ and F– E. coli cells
    C. Generalized transduction
    D. Transformation
    E. More than one of the above

B is correct.

Conjugations of F+ donor cells usually only transfer the F+ plasmid. The exception would be an F+ plasmid that has acquired a chromosomal gene in which case it would be designated an F′ plasmid.

401.   A site-specific recombination event would MOST likely occur during:
  A. The integration of a temperate bacteriophage into the bacterial chromosome
  B. Chromosomal inheritance from matings of Hfr by F– *E. coli* cells
  C. The transfer of the F+ plasmid
  D. The production of generalized transducing phage
  E. Incorporation of genes into the bacterial chromosome during bacterial transformations

A is correct.
Many temperate bacteriophages that integrate into the bacterial chromosome do so at a site containing specific base sequence.

For questions 402–405, match the restriction fragments that would result from digestion of the plasmid shown below.

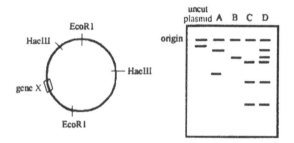

402.   Which lane on the agarose gel depicts the results anticipated from cutting the plasmid shown above with the restriction endonuclease EcoR1?

B is correct.
Since there are two EcoR1 restriction sites on the plasmid, one would normally expect to see two bands corresponding to the fragments. However, in this map, EcoR1 digestion will generate two fragments of nearly identical size because they are 180 degrees apart, which will appear as one band containing two fragments.

403. Which lane on the agarose gel represents the HaeIII digestion?

A is correct.
Since HaeIII has two sites on the plasmid it will generate two fragments and, based on their location, one will be larger than the other and separation will be good.

404.   Which lane corresponds to a double digest of the plasmid with both restriction endonucleases?

C is correct.
Normally you would look for four fragments but note that one of the EcoR1 fragments is cut in half by a HaeIII cut so this will result in two fragments of equal size and produce one band.

405.   Which lane would provide the lowest molecular weight fragment containing gene x following a double digest of the plasmid with both restriction end nucleases?

C is correct.
The top band from lane C contains gene x based on the size of the fragments produced from the double digest of the plasmid.

For questions 406–409, choose the single best answer.

406.   Which of the following genes are NOT carried on bacterial plasmids?
   A.   Antibiotic resistance genes
   B.   Genes for the synthesis of pili
   C.   Genes essential for the host cell growth
   D.   Genes that code for exotoxins
   E.   A variety of degradative enzymes

C is correct.
Plasmid DNA does not carry genes that are necessary for host survival such as genes required for their basic metabolic functions.

407.   All of the following statements regarding transposable genetic elements (transposons) are true EXCEPT:
   A.   The simplest of the transposons, IS elements, carry only a single gene that codes for the enzyme transposase
   B.   Complex transposons (Tn3) possess the enzyme resolvase which is responsible for site-specific recombination events
   C.   The direct base repeats found on the terminal ends of transposons are not part of the elements but rather are generated from the target DNA at insertion
   D.   Transposons can inactivate genes and cause mutations, but they do not activate or turn genes on
   E.   Antibiotic-resistance genes may become part of a transposon if an antibiotic-resistance gene should become flanked by two insertion sequence (IS) elements

D is correct.
In addition to behaving like mutagens by insertion into genes, some transposons are able to activate bacterial genes because they carry functional promotors.

408.   All the following statements regarding conjugation in *Streptococcus* is true EXCEPT:
   A.   Only certain plasmids can induce their transfer by conjugal union
   B.   Specific receptors (adhesins) are produced on the surface of the donor cells
   C.   Recipient cells lacking certain plasmids will secrete small peptides (sex pheromones) which cause the donor cells to adhere to the recipient cells
   D.   Acquisition of the conjugal plasmid causes the repression of the synthesis of the sex pheromones by the recipient cells
   E.   The mobilized chromosome in the donor cell is transferred to the recipient as a single strand of DNA

E is correct.
Conjugation in gram-positive bacteria results only in transfer of certain plasmids and has not been demonstrated to involve any chromosomal genes.

409. Type II restriction endonucleases (EcoR1) are the most desirable for use in recombinant DNA research and gene cloning because:
   A. Type II restriction-modification enzymes recognize a particular 4- or 6-base sequence
   B. Most type II enzymes cleave the DNA within or very near their recognition site
   C. Many type II enzymes cleave DNA in a staggered fashion leaving 3' or 5' overlapping 'sticky ends'
   D. Type II restriction endonucleases have separate enzymes for restriction and methylation and do not require ATP
   E. All of the above

E is correct.

For questions 410–413, match the numbered statement to the lettered genes or structures in the lactose operon being transcribed into polycistronic mRNA shown below.

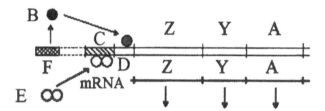

410. This protein is encoded by the *lac* regulatory gene and can interact with lactose or the operator gene.

B is correct.
The repressor protein may bind directly with the operator to shut-off transcription or may be inactivated by lactose.

411. The repressor protein binds to this specific DNA sequence making transcription by RNA polymerase impossible.

D is correct.
The operator sequence. In the absence of lactose (the inducer) the repressor protein is free to bind to the operator.

412. When lactose is the major carbon source, CAP-cAMP will bind to this sequence and cause maximum transcription of the genes.

C is correct.
The promotor sequences. When glucose levels are low, the cell produces cyclic AMP which binds to catabolite activator protein (CAP). This complex binds to the *lac* promotor maximizing transcription. Thus, both the presence of lactose and absence of glucose maximizes transcription.

413. In the absence of lactose, a repressor protein binds to this base sequence site and genes will not be transcribed.

D is correct.
Operator site. This accounts for the *lac* operon being a regulated structure (rather than constitutive). The absence of an inducer (allolactose molecules) allows a repressor protein to stop transcription.

Guide to other structures:
E.   RNA polymerase
F.   Regulatory gene

Pathogenic Bacteria

For questions 414–418, match the lettered toxin with the most appropriate numbered statement.

A. Endotoxin
B. Tetanus toxin
C. Botulism toxin
D. Pertussis toxin
E. Clostridial alpha toxin

414.   An adenosine diphosphate (ADP)-ribosyl transferase which effects the G regulatory protein leading to increased cAMP levels.

D is correct.
The pertussis toxin, like the cholera toxin and *Pseudomonas* exotoxin A, is also an ADP-ribosyl-transferase and one of its substrates is the G-protein which is involved in regulation of adenylate cyclase. The toxin causes an increase in cAMP which exaggerates the effects of cAMP-dependent processes. Peripheral lymphocytosis is one effect of the pertussis toxin.

415.   Causes fever and induces inflammation.

A is correct.
Endotoxin in low concentrations induces fever by acting on Kupffer cells and causes inflammation through the activation of complement. It also causes vasodilation and, at high concentrations, shock and intravascular coagulation.

416.   Causes muscle spasms.

B is correct.
Tetanus toxin (tetanospasmin) causes the inhibition of the transmitter release and normal inhibitory input resulting in the increase in resting tone and reflex spasms.

417.   Causes muscle paralysis.

C is correct.
The botulism neurotoxin prevents the release of the neurotransmitter acetylcholine and thus interferes with neurotransmission at peripheral cholinergic synapses

418.   Causes myonecrosis.

E is correct.
Lecithinase, the major toxin produced by *C. perfringens*, causes gas gangrene. The enzyme damages cell membranes and the muscle cells no longer react to stimuli.

For questions 419–421, match the lettered species of bacteria with the most appropriate numbered statement.

A. *Streptococcus pyogenes*
B. *Streptococcus agalactiae*
C. *Enterococcus faecalis*
D. *Streptococcus bovis*

419.   This organism has Lancefield group D antigen, grows in 6.5% NaCl, is part of normal enteric flora, and can cause urinary tract and cardiovascular infections.

C is correct.
E. faecalis, which is generally more resistant to antibiotics than the streptococci, grows in the presence of high concentrations of bile salts and NaCl.

420.   This organism produces streptococcal pyrogenic exotoxins (SPE) which are responsible for the symptoms of scarlet fever.

A is correct.
The pyrogenic exotoxins of this group A streptococcus have multiple effects including scarlet fever.

421.   This group D streptococcus will not grow in 6.5% NaCl, but it is usually sensitive to penicillin and has low virulence.

D is correct.
S. bovis is a non-enterococcal group D streptococcus which has been associated with endocarditis.

For questions 422–425, match the lettered species of bacteria with the most appropriate numbered statement.

   A. *Clostridium perfringens*
   B. *Neisseria gonorrhoeae*
   C. *Pseudomonas aeruginosa*
   D. *Escherichia coli*

422.   The organism which is the MOST likely to be responsible for a urinary tract infection.

D is correct.
E. coli is responsible for about 90% of all urinary tract infections in otherwise healthy persons.

423.   This organism is the MOST likely to cause conjunctivitis or eye infection in newborns if appropriate preventive measures are not taken.

B is correct.
It causes ophthalmia neonatorum, a purulent conjunctivitis in newborns. The disease is prevented by 1% silver nitrate, 1% tetracycline or 0.5% erythromycin eye ointments.

424.   This organism is commonly characterized by its O, K and H antigens and ability to ferment lactose.

D is correct.
E. coli serotyping is done using cell wall LPS, flagella H and surface polysaccharide K antigens.

425.   This organism is the most common bacterial pathogen to complicate the management of patients with cystic fibrosis.

C is correct.
Colonization of patients with cystic fibrosis (CF) by mucoid strains of *P. aeruginosa* has been associated with exacerbation of CF disease.

For questions 426–428, match the lettered bacterial product with the most appropriate numbered statement.

   A. Protein A
   B. p-toxin
   C. Enterotoxin C
   D. Alpha toxin

426.   This staphylococcal exoprotein is primarily responsible for the hemolysis surrounding colonies on blood agar plates at 37°C.

D is correct.
The staphylococcal alpha toxin is cytotoxic for a number of cells including erythrocytes. The toxin also disrupts the smooth muscle in blood vessels.

427. This is the most important toxin produced by *Clostridium perfringens* in myonecrosis.

D is correct.
The lecithinase or phospholipase C produced by all *C. perfringens* is also called alpha toxin.

428. This compound is associated with most strains of *Staphylococcus aureus* and is chemotactic, anticomplementary and antiphagocytic.

A is correct.
In addition to its unique affinity for the Fc receptor of immunoglobulins, protein A is also anticomplementary, a leukocyte chemoattractant, and inhibits opsonization and phagocytosis.

For questions 429–433, match the *Clostridium* species with its numbered description.

   A. *Clostridium tetani*
   B. *Clostridium botulinum*
   C. *Clostridium perfringens*
   D. *Clostridium difficile*

429. Normal microbial antagonism usually prevents disease by this organism.

D is correct.
C. difficile is part of the normal intestinal flora of healthy individuals. They cause disease only when alterations are made in their population such as by the use of antibiotics.

430. Responsible for a frequently fatal endometritis often seen after incomplete illegal abortions.

C is correct.
C. perfringens may infect the endometrium if it gains access to necrotic products of conception retained in the uterus.

431. Clinical symptoms of disease caused by this species include nausea, abdominal pain and diarrhea but NOT bloody diarrhea or fever.

C is correct.
C. perfringens enterotoxin food poisoning. Bloody diarrhea with fever is usually seen with infection by *C. difficile*.

432. Disease caused by this bacterium is prevented by immunization with toxoid.

A is correct.
Tetanus caused by the toxin produced by *C. tetani* is prevented by immunization with the toxoid.

433. An encapsulated, hemolytic species which produces four major and eight minor exotoxins.

C is correct.
C. perfringens produces several cytotoxins, the most important being alpha toxin which hydrolyzes lecithin and sphingomyelin.

For questions 434–436, match each bacterial species with its numbered description.

   A. *Bacteroides fragilis*
   B. *Pseudomonas aeruginosa*
   C. *Vibrio parahaemolyticus*
   D. *Bacillus cereus*

434. A gram-negative, motile bacillus that is one of the most common causes of infection from environmental contamination.

B is correct.
P. aeruginosa is an opportunistic inhabitant of the environment and commonly causes burns, wounds, urinary tract, skin, eye, ear and respiratory tract infections in compromised patients.

435.   Important for its role in the biodegradation of substances causing environmental pollution.

B is correct.
The same characteristics that allow *P. aeruginosa* to grow in some disinfectants allow them to degrade important environmental pollutants that would kill or inhibit the growth of other bacteria.

436.   Causes gastroenteritis associated with the consumption of raw seafood.

C is correct.
V. parahaemolyticus is a marine vibrio which is a major cause of gastroenteritis associated with raw seafood. The 'food poisoning' has a short incubation period of 24–48 hours, and is usually self-limiting.

For questions 437–439, match the lettered type of food poisoning with the most appropriate numbered statement.

A. Staphylococcus food poisoning
B. Salmonella food poisoning
C. *Clostridium perfringens* food poisoning
D. *Clostridium botulinum* food poisoning

437.   Consumption of this toxin results in the most highly fatal type of 'food poisoning'.

D is correct.
The toxins produced by *C. botulinum* (types A, B and E) are the most lethal of the 'food poisoning' bacteria; the mortality is 12–20%.

438.   This is the most common cause of food poisoning in the United States with symptoms appearing in about 6 hours.

A is correct.
Staphylococcus food poisoning caused by heat stable enterotoxins A and B can produce acute gastrointestinal symptoms within 2–5 hours after ingestion.

439.   Infection by this non-spore forming organism causes gastroenteritis with symptoms appearing in 24 hours.

B is correct.
Salmonella food poisoning produces symptoms in about 24 hours and is due to heat labile (LT) enterotoxin similar to *E. coli* and *V. cholerae* enterotoxins.

For questions 440–443, match the arthropod vector with the appropriate numbered pathogen.

A. Lice
B. Fleas
C. Ticks
D. Flies

440.   Transmission of *Yersinia pestis* to humans.

B is correct.
Sylvatic plague is transmitted by fleas infected with *Y. pestis*. The reservoirs for this organism in the United States include prairie dogs and rodents.

441.   Transmission of *Rickettsia rickettsii* to humans.

C is correct.
Rickettsia rickettsii causes Rocky Mountain spotted fever and is transmitted from rodents and dogs to humans by ticks.

442.   Transmission of *Francisella tularensis* to humans.

C is correct.
This pathogen, the causative agent of tularemia, is usually acquired from infected rabbits via direct contact with the carcass or via ticks.

443.   Transmission of *Ehrlichia chaffeensis* to humans.

C is correct.
Ehrlichia chaffeensis is transmitted to humans by ticks. Dogs or other wild or domestic animals are the source of the organism.

For questions 444–447, match the lettered growth medium used for isolation or differentiation with the appropriate numbered organism(s).

A. Medium with X and V factors
B. Blood agar containing tellurite
C. Thayer–Martin medium
D. MacConkey agar

444.   Required for growth of *Haemophilus influenzae.*

A is correct.
H. influenzae requires hematin and NAD for growth (X and V growth factors).

445.   Often used for isolation of *Neisseria gonorrhoeae.*

C is correct.
Thayer–Martin medium is a common medium for culturing *N. gonorrhoeae*. It contains vancomycin, an inhibitor of gram-positive organisms, and colistin and nystatin, inhibitors of some gram-negative bacteria and fungi, respectively.

446.   May be used for isolation of *Corynebacterium diphtheriae.*

B is correct.
On tellurite-containing medium *C. diphtheriae* colonies take on a characteristic dark appearance. A complex medium such as blood or coagulated serum (Loffler's) is required for primary isolation.

447.   A useful medium for the preliminary screening of enteric pathogens.

D is correct.
MacConkey agar is used for screening gram-negative organisms from stool, urine and other specimens. Lactose fermentation reactions are apparent on this medium.

For questions 448–451, match the lettered source of infection with the most appropriate bacterium.

A. Imported cheese made with non-pasteurized milk
B. Contaminated poultry products
C. Dog or cat bite
D. Man to man

448.   *Brucella melitensis.*

A is correct.
Brucellosis has been reduced to a few hundred cases per year in the United States and most are occupation exposures. The exception is usually small outbreaks traced to imported, unpasteurized dairy products.

449. *Salmonella typhimurium.*

B is correct.
Serotypes *S. typhimurium* and *S. enteritidis* are the most common causes of salmonella gastro-enteritis. Transovarially infected eggs and poultry are often the implicated vehicle of infection.

450. *Bordetella pertussis.*

D is correct.
Pertussis or whooping cough is spread by airborne droplets from patients in the early stages of illness.

451. *Pasteurella multocida.*

C is correct.
P. multocida is the most common type of infection acquired by the bite of a dog or cat.

For questions 452–456, match the lettered bacterial species with its description.

A. *Coxiella burnetii*
B. *Rickettsia prowazekii*
C. *Chlamydia psittaci*
D. *Ureaplasma urealyticum*

452. This micro-organism requires serum-enriched media for growth and produces a tiny 'fried egg' appearing colony.

D is correct.
Ureaplasma urealyticum, like the Mycoplasma, requires sterols provided by serum to maintain its membrane.

453. Distinguished by urease production and usually asymptomatic infection in women.

D is correct.
Ureaplasma urealyticum causes non-gonococcal urethritis in males and is usually asymptomatic in women.

454. A zoonosis, highly infectious and acquired through inhalation of aerosolized droppings from infected birds; rarely cultured because of risk of infection.

C is correct.
Chlamydia psittaci causes psittacosis and is usually acquired by inhalation of aerosolized dried bird droppings.

455. Transmitted by human body louse.

B is correct.
R. prowazekii causes louse-borne or epidemic typhus. The principal vectors are human body lice and, in sporadic cases in the United States, squirrel fleas.

456. Possesses a rigid outer membrane which is responsible for its shape.

D is correct.
Ureaplasma is one of two genera of prokaryotes that do not have a cell wall but rather a sterol-containing membrane that provides shape.

For questions 457–462, match the lettered bacterial species with its numbered description.

A. *Legionella pneumophila*
B. *Clostridium perfringens*
C. *Bacteroides fragilis*
D. *Bacillus cereus*

457. A gram-positive, anaerobic spore-forming bacterium which is a common cause of food poisoning.

B is correct.
C. perfringens, mainly type A but also a few types C and D strains, produces an enterotoxin. Clostridial food poisoning is usually the result of ingestion of contaminated meat products. Large numbers of contaminating organisms are required to produce clinical disease.

458. An obligate, anaerobe gram-negative, which is a major cause of disease involving anaerobic bacteria from endogenous sources.

C is correct.
B. fragilis is the most common cause of anaerobic infections from endogenous sources, although it comprises less than 1% of our colonic flora.

459. A facultative intracellular pathogen which multiplies in macrophages and causes Pontiac fever.

A is correct.
L. pneumophila, a self-limiting influenza-like infection.

460. A gram-negative, anaerobic bacillus resistant to bile salts. Subspecies may be recognized in part by their resistance to antibiotics.

C is correct.
B. fragilis is kanamycin, vancomycin and colistin resistant and its growth is stimulated by the addition of 20% bile in culture medium.

461. Ubiquitous distribution, with no person-to-person transmission proven. It is acquired by inhalation of aerosols. Culture medium must contain iron and L-cysteine.

A is correct.
L. pneumophila is nutritionally fastidious, requiring iron salts and L-cysteine in the growth media.

462. Growth is enhanced by the presence of algae and amebae; can withstand temperatures up to 55°C; diagnosed by direct immunofluorescence examination of respiratory secretions.

A is correct.
Legionella pneumophila is a parasite of protozoa and can be found in environments where amebae can act as a reservoir for virulent strains. Direct immunofluorescence using legionella-specific fluorescent antibody can be used for diagnosis.

For questions 463–468, match the bacterial species with its numbered description.

    A. *Fusobacterium fusiforme*
    B. *Clostridium difficile*
    C. *Clostridium tetani*
    D. *Clostridium botulinum*

463. Causes oral lesions in conjunction with a *Borrelia* spirochete.

A is correct.
F. fusiforme together with *Borrelia* spirochetes can cause an anaerobic, synergistic ulcerative infection of the gums, oral cavity or pharynx called Vincent's angina or trench mouth.

464. This anaerobic bacterium can cause an antibiotic-induced, pseudomembranous colitis.

B is correct.
C. difficile is responsible for most of this type of colitis. Antibiotic-associated diarrhea may be accompanied by the formation of a 'pseudo-membrane' composed of fibrin, leukocytes and necrotic colon cells.

465. The toxin produced by this micro-organism acts on the neuromuscular junction by inhibiting release of acetylcholine.

D is correct.
C. botulinum causes paralysis by blocking acetylcholine release.

466.   Its toxin acts by interfering with release of inhibitory neurotransmitters.

C is correct.
C. tetani produces tetanospasmin which blocks release of neurotransmitters for inhibitory synapses.

467.   Toxin produced by this organism is converted to toxoid and administered with DPT.

C is correct.
Tetanus toxoid is one of the components of the childhood vaccine. Booster with adult-type tetanus toxoid is recommended every 10 years after the age of 6 years.

468.   Colonization of an infant's colon causes poor muscle tone, lethargy and feeding problems.

D is correct.
Infants colonized with *C. botulinum* between the ages of 3 weeks and 8 months via dietary supplements will show the effects of absorption of the toxin.

For questions 469–475, match the bacterial species with its numbered description.

   A. *Mycoplasma pneumoniae*
   B. *Rickettsia rickettsii*
   C. *Chlamydia trachomatis*
   D. *Leptospira interrogans*

469.   The canicola serotype of this micro-organism is a frequent cause of disease by this species in the United States.

D is correct.
About 22 serotypes of *L. interrogans* are responsible for human infections in the United States. Serotype canicola which can infect dogs is a common source of leptospirosis in the United States.

470.   The L_1 subtype of this organism causes lymphogranuloma venereum.

C is correct.
Lymphogranuloma venereum is a chronic sexually transmitted disease caused by *C. trachomatis* serotypes L_1, L_2 and L_3.

471.   Produces characteristic 'inclusion bodies' in infected host cells.

C is correct.
Cytological examination of cell scraping will reveal the presence of inclusion bodies produced by the intracellular growth of *C. trachomatis*.

472.   Distinguished by its lack of peptidoglycan.

A is correct.
Mycoplasma pneumoniae does not have a cell wall and thus no peptidoglycan.

473.   Cold hemagglutinins produced in response to the glycolipids of the outer membrane of this infectious agent are helpful in diagnosis of the disease.

A is correct.
Non-specific reactions to the outer membrane glycolipids of *M. pneumoniae* produce IgM antibodies that bind the I antigen on the surface of human erythrocytes at 4°C.

474.   This micro-organism causes both epididymitis in males and conjunctivitis in infants of infected mothers.

C is correct.
C. trachomatis serotypes B and D-K.

475.   This organism is transovarially spread in tick vectors and is an obligate intracellular parasite.

B is correct.
R. rickettsii causes Rocky Mountain spotted fever. Its reservoir is wild rodents, it is spread (transovarily) in the progeny of the tick vector.

For questions 476 and 477, match the bacterial species with its numbered description.

   A. *Klebsiella pneumoniae*
   B. *Proteus mirabilis*
   C. *Salmonella enteritidis*
   D. *Vibrio cholerae*

476.   This species exhibits swarming motility and is commonly found in soil and sewage. Growth in urine will elevate pH which may be toxic to renal cells.

B is correct.
P. mirabilis produces large quantities of urease which splits urea into CO_2 and NH_3 elevating the pH of urine.

477.   Although non-invasive, this organism causes severe diarrhea and acidosis which can result in dehydration and shock.

D is correct.
V. cholerae produces enterotoxin that causes watery diarrhea and rapid fluid loss.

For questions 478–481, match each lettered bacterial species with its description.

   A. *Staphylococcus aureus*
   B. *Streptococcus pneumoniae*
   C. *Streptococcus agalactiae*
   D. *Streptococcus pyogenes*

478.   This species is exceptionally sensitive to lysis by deoxycholate and other bile salts.

B is correct.
S. pneumoniae undergoes rapid lysis when its autolysins are activated by exposure to bile.

479.   This species will grow in a nutrient broth supplemented with 6.5% NaCl, but it does not produce coagulase.

C is correct.
Unlike other streptococci, most isolates of *S. agalactiae* will grow in 6.5% NaCl.

480.   This organism can hydrolyze hippuric acid.

C is correct.
A preliminary identification of this group B streptococcus can be made by hydrolysis of hippurate.

481.   It can produce coagulase and ferments mannitol.

A is correct.
Staphylococcus aureus produces staphylocoagulase and ferments mannitol.

For questions 482–485, match the bacterial species with its numbered description.

   A. *Yersinia enterocolitica*
   B. *Campylobacter jejuni*
   C. *Vibrio* sp.
   D. *Mycobacterium tuberculosis*

482.   Selective isolation of this pathogen is aided by growth at 42°C in a microaerophilic atmosphere.

B is correct.
C. jejuni grows best at 42°C in an atmosphere of 5–7% O_2 and 5–10% CO_2.

483.   Isolation of this organism is enhanced by cold enrichment. Fecal specimens are mixed with saline and stored at 4°C.

A is correct.
Y. enterocolitica is metabolically active at lower temperatures which retard the growth of other species.

484.   This organism is not killed by treatment with 2% sodium hydroxide.

D is correct.
Decontamination of sputum specimens with 2% NaOH aids in the isolation *M. tuberculosis.*

485.   The isolation of this organism can be enhanced by its cultivation on an alkaline (pH 8.6) enrichment of peptone broth medium.

C is correct.
Many *Vibrio* sp. grow well in alkaline environments that inhibit most other contaminating bacteria. Growth of the halophilic vibrios, *V. parahaemolyticus, V. vulnificis,* etc., requires 1% sodium chloride supplementation to the media.

For questions 486–536, choose the single best answer.

486.   *Escherichia coli* K-1, *Haemophilus influenzae* type b, *Neisseria meningitidis* groups A, B and C, and *Streptococcus pneumoniae* are etiologic agents of bacterial meningitides in children. Which ONE of the following traits do they have in common?
    A. They are all part of the normal intestinal flora
    B. They are all usually resistant to penicillin G
    C. They are all gram-negative
    D. They all contain capsular polysaccharides

D is correct.
They all possess antiphagocytic polysaccharide capsules.

487.   Long-term carriage of the causative organism is most important in which of the following infections?
    A. Shigellosis
    B. *Campylobacter jejuni* infections
    C. Typhoid fever
    D. Salmonella gastroenteritis

C is correct.
Human carriers are the major source of *Salmonella typhi* which causes typhoid fever.

488.   Which of the following gonococcal infections is most common?
    A. Pelvic inflammatory disease
    B. Urethral strictures
    C. Gonococcal arthritis
    D. Opthalmia neonatorum

A is correct.
Ascending genital infection including pelvic inflammatory disease (PID) is reported in 10 to 20% of infected women.

489.   Which one of the following is MOST likely to allow a definitive diagnosis of typhoid fever?
    A. Culture of stool specimens for *Salmonella typhi* during the first week of illness
    B. Results of a Widal test for detection of anti-*S. typhi* O
    C. Culture of blood for *S. typhi* during the first week of illness
    D. Culture of urine for *S. typhi* during the first week of illness

C is correct.
Blood cultures should be positive and provide a definitive diagnosis in the early stages (first week) of typhoid fever.

490. Many infectious diseases are acquired by susceptible individuals through contact with persons who harbor the organism but are resistant to it. Which of the following diseases is NOT transmitted in this fashion?
   A. Neonatal streptococcus sepsis
   B. Diphtheria
   C. Infant botulism
   D. Meningococcal meningitis

C is correct.
Infant botulism is caused by the colonization of the gastrointestinal tract of young infants through food contaminated with *Clostridium botulinum*.

491. All of the following are true for the FTA-ABS test for syphilis EXCEPT:
   A. The patient's serum is used
   B. It is a direct immunofluorescent antibody test
   C. It requires an ultraviolet light microscope and darkened room to evaluate results
   D. The cultured Reiter strain of a non-pathogenic *Treponema* species is used for absorption of cross-reacting antibodies

B is correct.
This is an indirect immunofluorescence test because it employs a second antibody directed towards human IgG antibody.

492. Which of the following tests allows the earliest possible diagnosis of primary syphilis?
   A Darkfield examination of chancre fluid
   B. VDRL
   C. RPR
   D. FTA-ABS

A is correct.
T. pallidum spirochetes can be observed in chancre fluid before any reactive antibodies are produced.

493. A drop in antibody titer during antibiotic therapy for syphilis aids the physician in evaluating effectiveness of therapy. A drop in titer of which of the antibodies below is of most help in this respect?
   A. IgG to *T. pallidum*
   B. IgM to *T. pallidum*
   C. Reagin (antibody) to cardiolipin
   D. Antibody to Reiter strain of *T. pallidum*

C is correct.
VDRL and RPR tests both measure non-treponemal reagin antibodies (IgG and IgM). Unlike antibodies specific for the treponemal antigens, the reagin antibody titers drop with treatment and are therefore useful in monitoring therapy.

494. All of the following are gram-negative bacilli and opportunistic pathogens EXCEPT:
   A. *Escherichia coli*
   B. *Proteus vulgaris*
   C. *Serratia marcescens*
   D. *Lactobacillus acidophilus*

D is correct.
Lactobacillus acidophilus is a gram-positive bacillus. It is a non-pathogenic member of the human oral, gastrointestinal and vaginal flora.

495. Which of the following diseases is transmitted to man by urine from infected animals through cuts or abrasions in the skin?
   A. Sylvatic plague
   B. Tularemia
   C. Brucellosis
   D. Leptospirosis

D is correct.
Leptospira interrogans. This spirochete colonizes the renal tubes of many animal hosts and is shed in the urine in large numbers. There are approximately 22 serotypes of this species that can cause human disease.

496. Among infectious diseases which commonly present with an ulcer at the site of entry of the infecting agent are all of the following EXCEPT:
    A. Tularemia
    B. Chancroid
    C. Plague
    D. Brucellosis

D is correct.
Brucellosis is transmitted by ingestion of contaminated food or contact with infected animals. No ulcer develops at a site of entry.

497. Bacterial endocarditis often results from valvular colonization by organisms that are normal flora of the mouth and nasopharynx. Which of the following organisms is NOT commonly responsible for such infections?
    A. *Haemophilus parainfluenzae*
    B. *Streptococcus mutans*
    C. *Haemophilus aphrophilus*
    D. *Bordetella pertussis*

D is correct.
Bordetella pertussis is not a member of the normal flora in humans even though humans may have adequate immunity against disease caused by this organism.

498. Which organism is NOT correctly paired with a well-known inhibitory substance?
    A. *Streptococcus pneumoniae* – ethylhydrocupriene
    B. *Bordetella pertussis* – unsaturated fatty acids
    C. *Streptococcus pyogenes* – bacitracin
    D. *Staphylococcus aureus* – penicillin G

D is correct.
Almost all of strains of *Staphylococcus aureus* are resistant to β-lactamase-sensitive penicillins.

499. Which organism is NOT correctly paired with an appropriate culture medium?
    A. *Staphylococcus aureus* – mannitol salt agar
    B. *Haemophilus influenzae* – chocolate agar
    C. *Bordetella pertussis* – potato–glycerol–blood agar
    D. *Mycobacterium tuberculosis* – nutrient agar supplemented with rifampin

D is correct.
Mycobacterium tuberculosis is cultured on egg-based Lowenstein Jensen or Middlebrook media. Rifampin would inhibit growth.

500. Which of the following is NOT true for the VDRL and RPR tests?
    A. They employ *T. pallidum* as antigen
    B. They are subject to biologic false-positive reactions
    C. They frequently show false-negative results during tertiary syphilis
    D. They are helpful in evaluating a patient's response to therapy

A is correct.
The VDRL and RPR tests employ cardiolipin as antigens.

501. All of the following statements are true for *Listeria monocytogenes* EXCEPT:
    A. It is a facultative intracellular parasite
    B. Genital tract infection of the mother may lead to a condition known as granulomatis infantiseptica or to meningitis depending on whether infection occurs *in utero* or during passage through the birth canal
    C. This organism may cause disease such as meningitis in adults, especially in immunocompromised patients
    D. The organism is resistant to penicillin and most cases are nosocomial types of infections

D is correct.
L. monocytogenes is sensitive to penicillin or ampicillin and most infections are acquired by ingestion of contaminated food products or from asymptomatic human carriers.

502. Which of the following does NOT produce an IgA protease?
   A. *Neisseria gonorrhoeae*
   B. *Hemophilus influenzae*
   C. *Corynebacterium diphtheriae*
   D. *Staphylococcus aureus*

D is correct.
Staphylococcus aureus does not produce IgA protease.

503. Which of the following is NOT true for Lyme disease?
   A. It is caused by a spirochete which can be cultured
   B. It can be seen in blood specimens during febrile periods
   C. It is transmitted by *Ixodes* ticks
   D. The early stage of disease can be effectively treated with penicillin

B is correct.
The spirochete *B. burgdorferi* cannot be seen in blood specimens. *B. recurrentis* is visible in Giemsa or Wright stained specimens from relapsing fever patients.

504. Which of the following is NOT a correct association?
   A. *Chlamydia* – elementary bodies
   B. *Spirillum minor* – enterotoxin
   C. *Proteus vulgaris* antigens – Weil–Felix test
   D. *Streptococcus pneumoniae* – C reactive protein

B is correct.
Spirillium minor causes rat-bite fever which is characterized by chills, fever, rash and lymphadenopathy. No enterotoxins are associated with this organism.

505. Which of the following statements is NOT true for *Francisella tularensis*?
   A. It can be transmitted from animals to man by ticks
   B. It can be transmitted to man by contact with infected rabbits
   C. It can elicit both cell-mediated immune reactions and antibody formation in infected individuals
   D. It does not require specific nutrients for growth

D is correct.
Francisella tularensis requires cystine or cysteine for growth.

506. Which disease occurs in humans and other species?
   A. Syphilis
   B. Typhoid
   C. Q fever
   D. Gonorrhea

C is correct.
Q fever, caused by *Coxiella burnetii*, infects a large number of birds and animals in addition to humans.

507. Which of the following characteristics is NOT true regarding *Campylobacter jejuni*?
   A. It is one of the most common causes of infectious diarrhea
   B. It is microaerophilic and a curved gram-negative rod
   C. It is part of the normal intestinal flora of birds
   D. It may cause chronic gastric and peptic ulcers in humans

D is correct.
C. jejuni is not associated with an infectious type of gastric and peptic ulcers. *Helicobacter pylori* causes these types of infections.

508. Which of the following characteristics is NOT true for *Neisseria meningitidis*?
   A. It has an antiphagocytic polysaccharide capsule
   B. Group-specific anticapsular antibody is protective against infection
   C. Associated with the Waterhouse–Friedericksen syndrome
   D. Meningococcal bacteremia (meningococcemia) is the most common type of meningococcal infection

D is correct.
The most common form of meningococcal infection is acute purulent meningitis.

509.   Which of the following diseases is NOT usually transmitted by contact with healthy carriers but rather from contact with patients with the disease?
A. Meningococcal meningitis
B. Shigellosis
C. Diphtheria
D. Pneumonic plague

D is correct.
Pneumonic plague or pulmonary infection by *Yersinia pestis.*

510.   Which of the following statements is NOT true for *Shigella* species?
A. They can penetrate and multiply in intestinal epithelial cells but rarely penetrate beyond lamina propria
B. Laboratory diagnosis relies on isolation of organisms from the stool
C. Shigella are non-lactose-fermenting organisms
D. Like *Salmonella typhi, Shigella* species usually can be isolated from the blood of patients by blood culture obtained during the first week of the disease

D is correct.
Unlike salmonella, the shigella bacilli rarely penetrate beyond the mucosal layer and bacteremia is uncommon.

511.   Which of the following diseases is NOT considered to be a zoonosis?
A. Chancroid
B. Anthrax
C. Brucellosis
D. Leptospirosis

A is correct.
Chancroid is a sexually transmitted disease caused by *Haemophilus ducreyi.*

512.   Which of the following statements is NOT true for *Salmonella typhi?*
A. It penetrates and multiplies in lymphoid tissue (Peyer's patches) of the small intestine
B. It has a variety of animal reservoirs
C. It is present in blood during first week of disease at which time diagnosis can be made by blood culture
D. It is present in stools later in the disease at which time diagnosis is by stool culture

B is correct.
Salmonella serotype typhi is maintained by human carriage and not in animal reservoirs as are other *Salmonella* species.

513. Which of the following statements is NOT true for *Proteus mirabilis?*
A. It produces urease
B. When it infects the urinary tract, urine becomes alkaline
C. When streaked on blood agar, colonies produce waves of spreading growth due to 'swarming' motility
D. Its presence in feces is considered abnormal

D is correct.
Proteus mirabilis is an opportunistic pathogen found in the normal intestinal flora of man and animals.

514. Which of the following statements is NOT true for brucellosis?
   A. Infection of humans can be caused by at least three different species
   B. It produces enterotoxins that cause a severe diarrheal illness in humans
   C. Brucellosis of animals may pose a health hazard for veterinarians caring for sick animals
   D. Since pasteurization of milk, it is mainly an occupational disease

B is correct.
Brucellosis in humans is an infection primarily of the reticuloendothelial system. Virulent *Brucella* can enter and multiply in macrophages. Clinical manifestations are prolonged febrile periods with no enterotoxin or diarrhea.

515. Which of the following statements is NOT true with regard to pathogenic spore-forming organisms?
   A. The spores do not play a significant role in the epidemiology of their diseases
   B. The *Clostridia* are anaerobic spore formers which also produce potent exotoxins
   C. *Bacillus cereus* may cause food poisoning
   D. *Bacillus anthracis,* an aerobic spore former, has a polypeptide capsule composed of D-glutamic acid

A is correct.
Spores do play a role in establishing disease. They can protect the organisms from heat, O_2, dehydration, etc. until conditions favoring infection are present. Food poisoning can occur after spores survive brief heating or spores may germinate in necrotic tissue in the case of anaerobes.

516. Glycogen-containing inclusion bodies can be observed in infected cells of individuals with:
   A. Trachoma
   B. Psittacosis
   C. Gonorrhea
   D. Rocky Mountain spotted fever

A is correct.
The intracellular reproductive cycle of *Chlamydia trachomatis* serovars A, B, Ba and C cause trachoma. Inclusion containing elementary bodies and reticulate bodies can be seen in infected cells.

517. Which species can cause enteric fevers, septicemias or enterocolitis?
   A. *Salmonella* species
   B. *Klebsiella* species
   C. *Shigella* species
   D. *Escherichia* species

A is correct.
Salmonella species may cause enteric fevers, septicemias and enterocolitis.

518. All of the following gram-negative bacilli are members of the Enterobacteriaceae family and may be associated with nosocomial infections EXCEPT:
   A. *Citrobacter* species
   B. *Providencia* species
   C. *Campylobacter* species
   D. *Escherichia coli*

C is correct.
Campylobacter sp. are oxidase-positive, motile by means of polar flagella, and microaerophilic. They are not members of the Enterobacteriaceae family.

519. When a urine specimen is sent to the laboratory for bacterial culture, a bacterial count is done to indicate whether bacteria present are contaminants or the result of infection. What count in the urine would clearly indicate infection?
   A. 10^2 per ml
   B. 10^3 per ml
   C. 10^4 per ml
   D. 10^5 per ml or greater

D is correct.
Bacterial counts of 10^5 per ml or greater are clearly not contamination and indicate infection.

520.   Which of the following does NOT commonly present with an ulcer or lesion at the site of entry of the infecting agent?
   A. Tularemia
   B. Syphilis
   C. Leptospirosis
   D. Chancroid

C is correct.
Leptospira infections occur through small skin lesions, conjunctiva or most commonly, upper alimentary tract mucosa. No lesions occur at their site of entry.

521.   Bacteria which have NOT been cultured *in vitro* either on an agar medium or in cell culture are:
   A. *Mycoplasma* species
   B. *Chlamydia* species
   C. Rickettsial species
   D. *Treponema pallidum*

D is correct.
T. pallidum. Although it has shown brief growth in some primary cell cultures, it has not been sustained when passed in subculture and thus little is known of its metabolism.

522.   Which of the following diseases is NOT caused by spirochetes either alone or with other agents?
   A. Cat-scratch fever
   B. Vincent's angina
   C. Relapsing fever
   D. Lyme's disease

A is correct.
Cat-scratch fever is a febrile lymphadenitis caused by *Rochelimaea henselae*, a gram-negative bacilli.

523.   Which of the following is NOT true for *Streptococcus pyogenes*?
   A. Has M protein virulence factor
   B. Phage-typing distinguishes strains
   C. Has streptolysin O which is oxygen sensitive and antigenic
   D. Has lipoteichoic acid adherence factor

B is correct.
Phage-typing can be used to distinguish *Staphylococcus aureus* strains by their patterns of susceptibility and not *Streptococcus pyogenes*.

524.   An organism that causes urethritis with the greatest likelihood of ascending infection is:
   A. *E. coli*
   B. *Klebsiella*
   C. *Enterobacter*
   D. *Proteus*

D is correct.
The swarming motility of *Proteus* is believed to account for the high incidence of ascending urethral infections.

525.   Hemolytic uremic syndrome and hemorrhagic colitis have been most closely associated with:
   A. LT producing *E. coli*
   B. ST producing *E. coli*
   C. VT producing *E. coli*
   D. CFA/I (fimbriae) producing *E. coli*

C is correct.
The enterohemorrhagic *E. coli* produces the verotoxin VT or shiga-like toxin of *Shigella dysenteriae*.

526.   A sexually transmitted disease that produces a self-healing primary lesion followed by suppurated inguinal nodes that eventually discharge pus is caused by:
   A. *Mycoplasma*
   B. *Chlamydia trachomatis* serovars L1–L3
   C. *Ureaplasma urealyticum*
   D. *Neisseria gonorrhoeae*

B is correct.
Lymphogranuloma venereum caused by *C. trachomatis* serovars L1–L3.

527.   Which of the following toxins is NOT associated with virulent staphylococcus?
A. Leukocidin
B. LT enterotoxin
C. Exfoliative toxin
D. TSS toxin-1

B is correct.
The heat labile LT enterotoxin is produced by certain gram-negative enteric pathogens and not staphylococcus.

528.   The most reliable marker for virulence of *Staphylococcus* is:
A. Staphylokinase
B. Exotoxin C
C. Coagulase
D. β-lactamase

C is correct.
Coagulase bound to the cell wall (clumping factor) or cell-free coagulase-reacting factor (CRE) both convert fibrinogen to insoluble fibrin and are considered the best phenotypic indicator of *Staphylococcus* virulence.

529.   A component of the cell walls of most virulent strains of *Staphylococcus* that has affinity for binding the Fc receptor of certain immunoglobulins is:
A. Protein A
B. Teichoic acid
C. M protein
D. F protein

A is correct.
Protein A. It is sometimes used in serological tests as a non-specific carrier of antibodies directed against other antigens.

530.   Which of the following foods is LEAST likely to be the source of staphylococcal food poisoning?
A. Processed meats
B. Potato salad
C. Eggs and custard-filled pastries
D. Home-canned vegetables

D is correct.
While vegetables have been implicated in staphylococcal food poisoning, they represent the poorest growth medium of any of the foods listed. Since staphylococcal food poisoning is caused by toxin which requires growth of the bacteria, the other food substances account for most of the poisonings.

531.   Which of the following staphylococcal infections is always accompanied by the presence of another gram-positive cocci?
A. Scalded skin syndrome
B. Carbuncles
C. Impetigo
D. Endocarditis

C is correct.
Impetigo is usually caused by group A streptococcus alone but sometimes in combination with *S. aureus.*

532.   All of the following statements regarding staphylococcal enterotoxin are correct EXCEPT:
A. There are five serologically distinct toxins A-E and A is most commonly associated with illness
B. The enterotoxins are found only in certain strains of *S. aureus*
C. The enterotoxins are heat stable and resistant to denaturation at 100°C for 30 minutes
D. The enterotoxins are readily hydrolyzed by gastric and jejunal enzymes

D is correct.
Staphylococcal enterotoxins are not affected by gastric or jejunal enzymes.

533.   All of the following organisms can cause clinical syndromes similar to those caused by *S. aureus* infection EXCEPT:

A. Colitus – *Clostridium difficile*
B. Septic arthritis – *Neisseria gonorrhoeae*
C. Artificial valve endocarditis – *Staphylococcus epidermidis*
D. Tetanus – *Clostridium tetani*

D is correct.
No similarities exist between the clinical syndromes produced by *S. aureus* infections and *C. tetani*.

534.   All of the following organisms cause disease primarily in animals but can also infect humans EXCEPT:

A. *Coxiella burnetii*
B. *Leptospira interrogans*
C. *Borrelia burgdorferi*
D. *Salmonella typhi*

D is correct.
Enteric fever caused by *S. typhi* is maintained by human carriage.

535.   Which of the following organisms is NOT transmitted by an arthropod vector?

A. *Yersinia pestis*
B. *Borrelia burgdorferi*
C. *Rickettsia rickettsii*
D. *Mycoplasma pneumoniae*

D is correct.
M. pneumoniae is most commonly transmitted by aerosols and has no arthropod vector.

536.   All of the pathogens listed below gain entrance into the human body by the respiratory tract EXCEPT:

A. *Neisseria meningitidis*
B. *Salmonella enteritidis*
C. *Corynebacterium diphtheriae*
D. *Bordetella pertussis*

B is correct.
Salmonella enteritidis infects through the gastro-intestinal tract.

For questions 537 and 538, choose the single best answer based on the figure below, which shows a smear from the vagina of a normal 23-year-old woman without any apparent infection. The major organism is a gram-positive bacillus or streptobacillus.

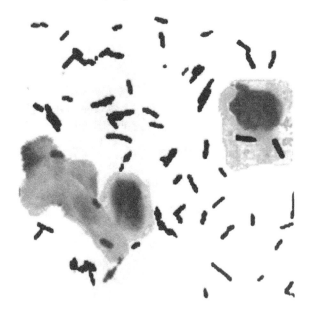

537. The MOST likely organism in the vaginal smear is:
    A. *Erysipelothrix rhusiopathiae*
    B. *Lactobacillus acidophilus*
    C. *Listeria monocytogenes*
    D. *Moraxella lacunata*

B is correct.
Lactobacilli are members of the normal human oral, gastrointestinal and vaginal flora.

538. The primary metabolic product of the predominant human vaginal flora is:
    A. Ethanol
    B. Pyruvic acid
    C. Lactic acid
    D. CO_2

C is correct.
The normal vaginal flora actively ferments carbohydrates, forming lactic acid as the primary metabolic product, and aids in maintaining an acidic environment.

For questions 539 and 540, choose the single best answer based on the figure below, which depicts gram-negative diplococci within polymorphonuclear leukocytes from a smear of a urethral exudate.

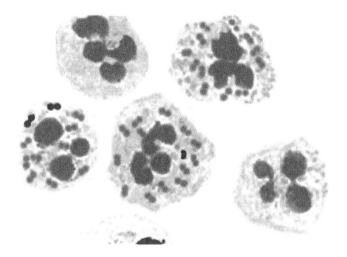

539. The follow-up diagnostic procedure would MOST likely be based on the assumption that the observed organism is:
    A. *Chlamydia trachomatis*
    B. *Neisseria gonorrhoeae*
    C. *Calymmatobacterium granulomatis*
    D. *Haemophilus ducreyi*

B is correct.
It appears as a typical intracellular gram-negative diplococcus in polymorphonuclear leukocytes.

540. In the case of gonococcal urethritis, which of the following organisms is most likely to co-infect with *N. gonorrhoeae*?
    A. *Chlamydia trachomatis*
    B. *Haemophilus ducreyi*
    C. *Treponema pallidum*
    D. *Staphylococcus aureus*

A is correct.
Chlamydia trachomatis is the most common sexually transmitted bacterial disease and co-infections with *N. gonorrhoeae* are common. The same treatment will clear up both infections.

For questions 541–544, match the lettered bacterial species with the appropriate numbered description.

A. *Ehrlichia chaffeensis*
B. *Vibrio vulnificus*
C. *Listeria monocytogenes*
D. *Haemophilus aegyptius*
E. *Streptococcus pneumonia*

541.   This small gram-negative rod requires hemin and NAD for growth. It causes conjunctivitis (pinkeye).

D is correct.
H. aegyptius is also known as *H. influenzae* type III because of its close relationship with *H. influenzae*. It is highly contagious and new variants have recently been isolated from the blood of patients with Brazilian purpuric fever, an often life-threatening disease.

542.   This gram-negative bacterium causes gastroenteritis. It is a free-living marine organism which is not associated with pollution and is commonly found in the Gulf of Mexico.

B is correct.
This vibrio is associated with the consumption of raw oysters. It carries a high mortality rate in persons with compromised immune systems or pre-existing liver disease.

543.   This organism is transmitted by ticks. It produces a disease which resembles rickettsial infections. However, there is no rash and the patients are negative for the Weil–Felix test.

A is correct.
Clinical symptoms include malaise, fever and headache.

544.   A gram-negative rod that infects the blood and nervous system. Transmission is through contact with infected soil and animal food products such as cheese. High monocyte counts are usually observed in infected individuals.

C is correct.
Listeria monocytogenes may clinically resemble meningitis and if contracted during pregnancy may result in miscarriage.

For questions 545 and 546, choose the single best answer based on the figure below, which is a micrograph of gram-stained sputum of a patient with pneumonia. The bacteria appear as gram-positive, lancet-shaped diplococci.

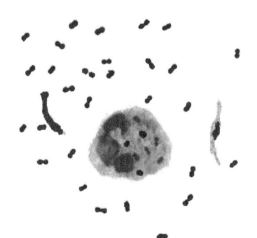

545. The MOST likely organism in the sputum smear is:
    A. *Klebsiella pneumoniae*
    B. *Haemophilus influenzae*
    C. *Streptococcus pneumoniae*
    D. *Viridans* streptococci

C is correct.
S. pneumoniae is consistent with the morphology and gram stain and a common cause of pneumonia.

546. Which laboratory test is routinely used to confirm *S. pneumoniae* in the patient's sputum?
    A. Quellung test
    B. Optochin susceptibility or bile solubility
    C. Detection of specific antigens in body fluids
    D. All of the above

B is correct.
While all of the tests listed have the potential to confirm the organism as *S. pneumoniae*, the laboratory would use the optochin or bile tests to confirm the species.

Mycology

For questions 547–575, choose the single best answer.

547. Many fungal infections are the result of spore inhalation. One which is usually NOT contracted in this manner is:
    A. Histoplasmosis
    B. Blastomycosis
    C. Coccidioidomycosis
    D. Sporotrichosis

D is correct.
Sporotrichosis is caused by *Sporothrix schenckii* and is introduced into the subcutaneous layer of the skin by traumatic implantation, i.e. thorns.

548. A mycotic infection which is similar to pulmonary tuberculosis in that it is seen in primary and reinfection forms, with multiple calcified areas in the lungs, and specific delayed hypersensitivity skin test, is:
    A. Candidiasis
    B. Sporotrichosis
    C. Histoplasmosis
    D. Aspergillosis

C is correct.
Histoplasma capsulatum can grow within macrophages, and thereby escape normal defense mechanisms and cause progressive, destructive lesions similar to tuberculosis.

549. The india ink mount is most useful for establishing a diagnosis of:
    A. Nocardiosis
    B. Blastomycosis
    C. Histoplasmosis
    D. Cryptococcosis

D is correct
A rapid diagnosis of cryptococcal meningitis can often be made by examination of an India ink preparation of cerebrospinal fluid because of the large capsule surrounding *Cryptococcus neoformans*.

550. The fungistatic or fungicidal activity of amphotericin B is related to its ability to:
    A. Inhibit cell wall synthesis
    B. Inhibit protein synthesis
    C. Disrupt the cell membrane
    D. Destroy mitochondria

C is correct.
Amphotericin B binds to ergosterol-containing membranes where it forms pores which increase membrane permeability.

551. Which disease is often associated with dust from bird or bat manure?
    A. North American blastomycosis
    B. Histoplasmosis
    C. Both of the above
    D. Neither of the above

B is correct.
Histoplasma capsulatum grows well in soil rich in excreta from birds due to its high nitrogen content. Natural infection does occur in bats.

552.   Which of the following organisms has a predilection for lymphatic tissue?
   A. Chromomycosis etiologic agents
   B. *Sporothrix schenckii*
   C. *Blastomyces dermatitidis*
   D. *Coccidioides immitis*

B is correct.
Sporothrix schenckii may cause lymphocutaneous sporotrichosis characterized by nodular and ulcerative lesions along lymphatics.

553.   Which organism grows in tissues or cultures at 37°C as a thick-walled budding yeast with only a single bud per cell, but in cultures at room temperature grows as a mycelium with lateral, rounded conidia along the hyphae?
   A. *Coccidioides immitis*
   B. *Histoplasma capsulatum*
   C. *Blastomyces dermatitidis*
   D. *Sporothrix schenkii*

C is correct.
Blastomyces dermatitidis, a typical dimorphic fungus, has both yeast and filamentous forms as do most human systemic fungal pathogens.

554.   The most useful laboratory test for distinguishing *Candida albicans* from similar yeast forms is:
   A. Germ-tube test
   B. Resistance to cycloheximide
   C. Hemagglutination test
   D. Uptake of neutral red

A is correct.
Blastospores of *C. albicans* produce hyphal outgrowths or germ tubes within 2–3 hours of incubation in serum at 37°C.

555.   The medically important fungi are identified principally on the basis of:
   A. Staining properties
   B. Biochemical activity
   C. Nutritive requirements
   D. Reproductive structures

D is correct.
Reproductive structures of medically important fungi usually differ enough to lead to their identification.

556.   The following organism is endemic in the San Joaquin Valley in California:
   A. *Blastomyces dermatitidis*
   B. *Cryptococcus neoformans*
   C. *Coccidioides immitis*
   D. *Histoplasma capsulatum*

C is correct.
Coccidioides immitis causes coccidiodomycosis, also called Posada's disease, San Joaquin Valley fever or desert rheumatism.

557.   Which of the following is NOT a characteristic of *Histoplasma capsulatum*?
   A. It is associated with birds
   B. It generally produces flu-like symptoms in man
   C. It causes infection resulting in pulmonary coin lesions
   D. It produces a potent exotoxin

D is correct.
H. capsulatum does not produce any exotoxin; very few pathogenic fungi do. *Aspergillus*, an opportunistic fungus, is the exception.

558.   The important diagnostic feature of *Blastomyces dermatitidis in vivo* is:
   A. Coenocytic hyphae
   B. Hyphae less than 1 μm in diameter
   C. Granule formation
   D. Broad-based yeast cells

D is correct.
The broad-based budding yeast cells in infected tissue are a good diagnostic feature of *B. dermatitidis*.

559. Ringworm and athlete's foot are examples of:
    A. Fungal infections which are treated with streptomycin
    B. Infections caused by *Candida*
    C. Systemic mycoses
    D. Superficial mycoses

D is correct.
Infections of the outermost layers of the skin and hair are caused by several species of dermatophytes.

560. What are fungal spores formed as a result of hyphal cell fragmentation called?
    A. Chlamydospores
    B. Arthrospores
    C. Blastospores
    D. Conidia

B is correct.
Arthrospores such as those produced by *Coccidioides immitis.*

561. *Cryptococcus neoformans* can be found growing most often in:
    A. Water
    B. Soil containing pigeon feces
    C. Chicken feces
    D. Desert soils

B is correct.
There is a close relationship to the habitats of pigeons and *C. neoformans*, but it does not naturally infect the bird.

562. The etiologic agent of which of these infections is dimorphic?
    A. Sporotrichosis
    B. Blastomycosis
    C. Both of the above
    D. Neither of the above

C is correct.
Both fungi have a parasitic yeast phase and saprophitic 'mold' form.

563. Which of the following structures is NOT the result of sexual reproduction?
    A. Ascospore
    B. Basidiospore
    C. Chlamydoconidia
    D. Zygospore

C is correct.
Chlamydoconidia are asexual structures that develop within the hyphae. Asexual reproductive elements are called conidia. Those produced sexually are called spores.

564. Dermatophytes have a particular affinity for skin and related tissues because of the presence in the tissue of:
    A. Carotene
    B. Normal bacterial flora
    C. Keratin
    D. Lipids

C is correct.
These fungi are also referred to as keratinophilic because they possess keratinase which allows them to utilize keratin as a substrate.

565. What is the MOST probable port of entry for the fungus causing aspergillosis?
    A. Puncture wound
    B. Blood
    C. Lungs
    D. Gastrointestinal tract

C is correct.
Aspergillus is extremely common in the environment and is usually acquired by inhalation.

566. Yeasts reproduce asexually by means of:
    A. Conidia
    B. Sporangiospores
    C. Macroconidia
    D. Blastoconidia

D is correct.
Blastoconidia. Sexual reproduction in yeast leads to the formation of ascospores.

567. *Cryptococcus neoformans* has a particular predilection for the:
   A. Brain and meninges
   B. Lung
   C. Skin
   D. Hair

A is correct.
The clinical entity most often seen with *C. neoformans* is cryptococcal meningitis.

568. What are conidia in the fungi?
   A. Sexual spores
   B. Undifferentiated bits of hyphae
   C. Asexual spores
   D. Discharged from gills of mushrooms

C is correct.
Conidia are asexual reproductive bodies of fungi.

569. The MOST common factor predisposing to systemic *Candida albicans* infection is:
   A. Diabetes
   B. Intravenous heroin use
   C. Long-term antibiotic therapy
   D. AIDS

C is correct.
Prolonged use of broad-spectrum antibiotic therapy is the most common underlying cause of disseminated candidiasis. AIDS patients commonly develop oropharynx or upper gastro-intestinal infections but rarely systemic disease.

570. A dimorphic fungus will have which of the following forms?
   A. Mycelium in tissue and mycelium in soil
   B. Yeast in tissue and mycelium in soil
   C. Yeast in tissue and yeast in soil
   D. Mycelium in tissue and yeast in soil

B is correct.
Yeast forms are found in tissue at 37ºC. Mycelium or mold forms are found in soil and in culture media at 25º C.

571. Which of the following patients should be isolated to prevent possible spread of their fungal infection to another patient?
   A. A female with oral candidiasis
   B. An adult with pulmonary cavitary coccidioidomycosis
   C. A 6-year-old child with *Microsporum canis* infection of the scalp
   D. A 10-year-old child with cutaneous sporotrichosis

C is correct.
The dermatophytes are the only fungi that can be transferred from man to man.

572. The formation of pseudohyphae is characteristic of which of the following?
   A. *Histoplasma capsulatum*
   B. *Coccidioides immitis*
   C. *Candida* spp.
   D. *Cryptococcus neoformans*

C is correct.
Candida spp. produce pseudohyphae.

573. Which of the following produce only yeast forms when grown on blood agar plates at either room temperature or at 37ºC?
   A. *Blastomyces dermatitidis*
   B. *Coccidioides immitis*
   C. *Cryptococcus neoformans*
   D. *Histoplasma capsulatum*

C is correct.
Cryptococcus neoformans, unlike other systemic mycotic agents, does not have a dimorphic asexual phase. Yeast forms are observed at 25 and 37ºC.

574.   Which of the following produce large tuberculate macroconidia in culture on plates incubated at room temperature?
   A.   *Blastomyces dermatitidis*
   B.   *Coccidioides immitis*
   C.   *Cryptococcus neoformans*
   D.   *Histoplasma capsulatum*

D is correct.
Tuberculate microconidia are formed by *H. capsulatum* at 25°C.

575.   Endospherules may be observed in the tissues or fluids of patients infected with:
   A.   *Blastomyces dermatitidis*
   B.   *Coccidioides immitis*
   C.   *Cryptococcus neoformans*
   D.   *Sporothrix schenckii*

B is correct.
Endospherules or spherules are endospore-filled structures that develop in tissue infected by *C. immitis*

For questions 576–578, match the lettered disease with its causative agent.

   A.   Candidiasis
   B.   Blastomycosis
   C.   Coccidiodomycosis
   D.   Cryptococcosis

576.   This disease is caused by a gram-positive fungus that produces chlamydospores when grown on cornmeal agar.

A is correct.
Cornmeal agar is a useful culture medium to aid in the identification of *Candida* by colonial morphology. Although too large to be bacteria, the yeast phase of *Candida* spp. stain gram-positive.

577.   The development of oral infections with this organism should alert physicians to the possibility of immunodeficiency.

A is correct.
Thrush or oral candidiasis occurs at a high frequency in individuals with T lymphocyte immunodeficiencies even though the infections may be superficial.

578.   Large encapsulated budding yeast cells can often be observed in India ink preparations of cerebrospinal fluids.

D is correct.
Cryptococcus neoformans has a very large polysaccharide capsule and meningitis is the most commonly recognized form of cryptococcal disease.

For questions 579 and 580, match the disease with its causative organism.

   A.   Superficial mycoses
   B.   Cutaneous mycoses
   C.   Systemic mycoses
   D.   Subcutaneous mycoses

579.   Species or strains of zoophilic origins tend to cause more inflammatory lesions than those of anthropophilic origins.

A is correct.
Superficial mycoses such as ringworm infections of the skin called tinea corporis caused by a dermatophyte of animal origin such as *Microsporum canis*, will induce a more inflammatory lesion than a species of human origin such as *M. audouinii.*

580. Most infections are acquired by the inhalation of spores.

C is correct.
Systemic mycoses usually start with a pulmonary infection from inhalation of infectious bodies and may then disseminate to other organs.

For questions 581–583, match the lettered fungal filamentious and yeast forms in the figure with the appropriate numbered description.

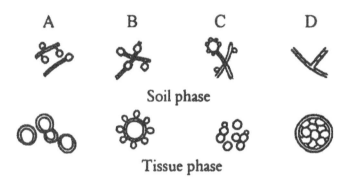

581. The microscopic morphology of this fungal pathogen resembles that of *Histoplasma capsulatum*.

C is correct.
The mold phase shows characteristic tuberculate macroconidia while the tissue phase is usually seen as yeast forms filling a macrophage.

582. Which figure best depicts *Coccidioides immitis*?

D is correct.
The resistant, infectious arthrospores and the thick-walled spherules found in tissue allow for easy identification of this fungal pathogen.

583. Causes North American blastomycosis.

A is correct.
The thick-walled, broad-based budding yeast form is characteristic of *Blastomyces dermatitidis*.

Parasitology

For questions 584–587, match the lettered parasite with the appropriate numbered description.

- A. *Mycobacterium avium–intracellulare*
- B. *Toxoplasma gondii*
- C. *Pneumocystis carinii*
- D. *Nocardia asteroides*
- E. More than one of the above

584. The most common cause of opportunistic infections in AIDS patients.

C is correct.
Although subclinical infections appear to be widespread, immunocompromised hosts have a high mortality rate from pneumonia caused by *P. carinii*.

585. The domestic cat is the definitive host for this protozoan parasite and although subclinical infections are very common, immunosuppressed individuals are at high risk.

B is correct.
Immunosuppressed individuals may become diseased from latent infections as well as primary infection. *T. gondii* may give rise to several types of infections including congenital infections.

586. An acid-fast organism, widespread in nature in soil and water.

E is correct.
Both *Nocardia asteroides* and strains belonging to the *Mycobacterium avium–intracellulare* complex are found in soil and water, have low invasiveness, and usually cause subclinical infections in normal individuals. They are a common cause of disease in immunosuppressed individuals.

587. Skin tests indicate a very high incidence of inapparent infections in normal humans; however, this organism causes very high morbidity and mortality in immunodeficient individuals.

A is correct.
The MAC complex produces disease in animals, birds, insects, etc. and is a very common infection in AIDS patients. Healthy individuals appear to be resistant to clinical infection.

For questions 588–592, match the numbered statement with the most appropriate lettered pathogen.

  A. *Entamoeba histolytica*
  B. *Entamoeba coli*
  C. *Naegleria fowleri*
  D. *Acanthamoeba* sp.
  E. More than one of the above

588. This non-pathogenic protozoan commonly parasitizes the human gastrointestinal tract. It is important because it must be differentiated from pathogenic amebae.

B is correct.
Entamoeba coli can be microscopically differentiated from *E. histolytica* by its 1–8 nuclei and the splintered, frayed ends on its chromatid bars in the cysts. The trophozoite has coarse, clumped peripheral nuclear chromatin. Compare this with the 1–4 nuclei and fine dispersed chromatin in *E. histolytica*.

589. This free-living ameba is an opportunistic pathogen that can cause a rapidly fatal primary amebic meningo-encephalitis.

C is correct.
Naegleria fowleri infections usually occur when individuals are exposed by swimming in contaminated streams or lakes. The ameba enters the body through mucous membranes of the nose and follows the olfactory tract to the brain. Patients show Kernig's sign and trophozoites are present in spinal fluid.

590. This organism is the most common cause of amebic dysentery. Symptoms include abdominal pain, cramping, colitis and diarrhea. Characteristic colonic ulcers may be observed by sigmoidoscopic examination.

A is correct.
Entamoeba histolytica has a world-wide prevalence of 10–15% and in the United States, 1–2%. Sources of infection are food and contaminated water by asymptomatic carriers and oral–anal sexual practices.

591.   This organism can cause granulomatous amebic encephalitis primarily in immunocompromised individuals or keratitis usually associated with trauma to the eye or improper cleaning of contact lenses.

D is correct.
Similar to *Naegleria*, this free-living organism is acquired by contact with contaminated soil dust and water. Diagnosis is by microscopic observation in tissue, and the organism can be cultured.

592.   Liver abscess may result from invasion of the blood stream by the trophozoites.

A is correct.
Both low virulent and invasive strains of *E. histolytica* have been identified. The latter are more likely to cause extra-intestinal amebiasis.

For questions 593–598, match the numbered statement with the most appropriate lettered pathogen.

    A. *Giardia lamblia*
    B. *Dientamoeba fragilis*
    C. *Trichomonas vaginalis*
    D. *Balantidium coli*
    E. More than one of the above

593.   This is not an intestinal protozoan.

C is correct.
Trichomonas vaginalis causes urogenital infections.

594.   This ciliated protozoan is commonly contracted by people in contact with swine and living under substandard hygienic conditions. Infection is characterized by ulceration of the intestinal mucosa leading to tenesmus, abdominal pain and watery stools without blood or pus.

D is correct.
Microscopic examination of the feces from infected patients reveals cysts and very large ciliated trophozoites. *B. coli* is the only ciliated parasite found in humans.

595.   Sexual transmission by asymptomatic hosts is the primary mode of infection by this organism.

C is correct.
Men are the primary asymptomatic carriers of *T. vaginalis* and serve as reservoirs of infection for women who are also frequently asymptomatic. However, they may develop urethritis or prostatitis.

596.   This protozoan exists only in the trophozoite form.

E is correct.
Trichomonas vaginalis and *Dientamoeba fragilis* have no cyst forms.

597.   The trophozoites attach to the intestinal villi by a prominent ventral sucking disk. Clinical symptoms range from none (50%) to severe malabsorption.

A is correct.
Diarrhea may include steatorrhea. Blood or pus in stools is rare.

598.   This flagellate has a world-wide distribution; ecologically it ranges from remote wilderness areas due to animal reservoirs, to highly endemic areas where it is spread by contaminated food and water or person-to-person contact.

A is correct.
In addition to endemic disease, major outbreaks occur in day-care centers, institutions and among homosexual populations.

For questions 599 and 600, match the numbered statement with the most appropriate lettered pathogen.

    A. *Plasmodium vivax*
    B. *Plasmodium ovale*
    C. *Plasmodium malariae*
    D. *Plasmodium falciparum*
    E. All of the above

599. The most prevalent of the plasmodia, it also has the widest geographical distribution.

A is correct.
Plasmodium vivax causes benign tertian malaria and disease extends into the temperate regions.

600. Syndromes caused by infections with this plasmodium are termed malignant tertian malaria and/or black water fever. It has a distinctive sausage-shaped mature gametocyte.

D is correct.
The clinical symptoms result from kidney damage (black water fever) or intestinal involvement that causes vomiting and diarrhea (malignant tertiary malaria).

For questions 601–604, match the numbered statement with the most appropriate lettered pathogen.

    A. *Cryptosporidium* sp.
    B. *Microsporidia* sp.
    C. *Toxoplasma gondii*
    D. *Pneumocystis carinii*
    E. More than one of the above

601. This intracellular coccidian parasite is acquired by ingestion of oocysts from contamination by cat feces or cysts in undercooked meats. The development of the tachyzoite form causes tissue damage, and congenital infections carry very high morbidity and mortality rates.

C is correct.
Immunocompromised individuals (AIDS, organ transplant recipients, etc.) show severe symptoms which are commonly neurological. ELISA tests for IgM antibodies are useful for non-AIDS patients.

602. This organism is closely related to the fungi and is transmitted by respiratory droplets and close contact. Infections commonly cause interstitial pneumonitis and the organism can usually be observed in bronchoalveolar lavage fluid.

D is correct.
Pneumocystis carinii pneumonia, previously associated primarily with malnourished and institutionalized children, develops in 80–90% of AIDS patients.

603. This primitive intracellular parasite causes chronic diarrhea in immunocompromised patients. In some AIDS patients, disseminated disease may occur. Diagnosis can be made by observing characteristic oocysts in stool specimens which are stained using a modified acid-fast method.

A is correct.
Cryptosporidium is distributed world-wide, and there is zoonotic spread from a wide variety of animals by the fecal–oral route. Specimens may be stained using a modified acid-fast method.

604. An obligate intracellular pathogen which produces characteristic spores that can be visualized in biopsy material with various stains including the gram stain (gram-positive). The organism causes a disseminated disease capable of infecting every organ in the body.

B is correct.
Five genera of this phylum infect man. They lack mitochondria and several other eukaryotic organelles. The reservoir of infection is a wide range of invertebrate and vertebrate animals. Spores are shed in urine and feces of infected individuals.

For questions 605–609, match the lettered protozoan in the figure with its numbered description.

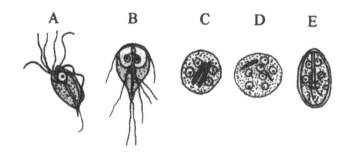

605.   The cyst of *Entamoeba coli.*   D is correct.

606.   The trophozoite of *Giardia lamblia.*   B is correct.

607.   The cyst of *Entamoeba histolytica.*   C is correct.

608.   The cyst of *Giardia lamblia.*   E is correct.

609.   The trophozoite of *Trichomonas hominis.*   A is correct.

For questions 610–615, match the lettered mode of transmission with the numbered nematode species.

    A. Hand to mouth
    B. Ingestion of human feces
    C. Skin penetration
    D. Consumption of undercooked pork
    E. Skin penetration and auto-infection

610.   *Ascaris lumbricoides* (round worm).

B is correct.
Human feces-contaminated soil in heavy endemic regions. Migration of the worms to the bile duct and liver, and other tissue damage accounts for most of its pathology.

611.   *Trichinella spiralis.*

D is correct.
A common parasitic disease in the United States. Pathology is associated with larval migrations, and heavy infections carry high morbidity and mortality rates.

612.   *Trichuris trichiura* (whip worm).

B is correct.
Usually asymptomatic, heavy worm burdens cause bloody diarrhea, appendicitis and bacterial infections due to penetration of the intestinal mucosa.

613. *Strongyloides stercoralis* (threadworm).

E is correct.

Fecal contaminated soil and auto-infection. Filariform larvae can penetrate intestines and circulate through the lungs back into the intestines. Free-living adults are found in soil and produce infective larvae forms similar to hookworm. Sexual transmission also occurs.

614. *Enterobius vermicularis* (pinworm).

E is correct.

Skin penetration is the most common route of infection although hand to mouth is also possible. Enterobiasis is usually asymptomatic but may cause pruritis and bacterial infection in allergic hosts. Genitourinary complications may also occur.

615. *Necator americanus* (hookworm).

C is correct.

Infective larvae in soil penetrate the skin. Symptoms may include allergic reactions, skin rash, pneumonitis, diarrhea, anemia and emaciation.

For questions 616–620, match the lettered disease with the numbered causative agent and vector for transmission.

    A. Visceral leishmaniasis (Kala-azar fever)
    B. Mucocutaneous leishmaniasis (American leishmaniasis, chiclero ulcer)
    C. Cutaneous leishmaniasis (oriental sore)
    D. American trypanosomiasis (Chagas' disease)
    E. African trypanosomiasis (sleeping sickness)

616. *Leishmania donovani* – sand flies.

A is correct.

617. *Trypanosoma cruzi* – kissing bug.

D is correct.

618. *Trypanosoma brucei* – tsetse fly.

E is correct.

619. *Leishmania tropica* – sand flies.

C is correct.

620. *Leishmania braziliensis* – sand flies.

B is correct.

For questions 621–627, match the lettered egg in the figure with the appropriate numbered pathogen.

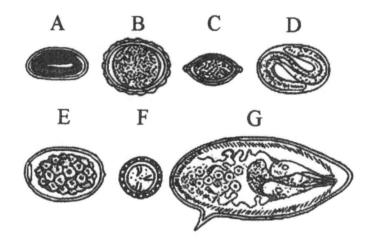

621. *Ancylostoma duodenale* or *Necator americanus* (hookworms).

D is correct.
A bluntly ovoid egg with a transparent shell. The species cannot be differentiated.

622. *Ascaris lumbricoides* (roundworm).

B is correct.
A rough, thick-shelled egg.

623. *Trichuris trichiura* (whipworm).

C is correct.
A barrel-shaped egg with polar plugs.

624. *Enterobus vermicularis* (pinworm).

A is correct.
An asymmetrical egg containing a fully developed larva.

625. *Schistosoma mansoni.*

G is correct.
A thin shell with a prominent lateral spine.

626. *Diphyllobothrium latum* (fish tapeworm).

E is correct.
Eggs are operculated, with a knob on the bottom of the shell.

627. *Taenia* sp. (beef or pork tapeworm).

F is correct.
Thick walled, spherical and containing hooklets. Species cannot be differentiated at this stage.

For questions 628–632, match the lettered species of cestodes with their numbered reservoir of infestation.

  A. *Taenia solium*
  B. *Taenia saginata*
  C. *Diphyllobothrium latum*
  D. *Echinococcus* sp.
  E. *Hymenolepsis* sp.

628. Raw beef.

B is correct.

629.   Raw fish.   C is correct.

630.   Insects, rodents and auto-infections.   E is correct.

631.   Canines and cats.   D is correct.

632.   Raw pork.   A is correct.

For questions 633–635, match the lettered row showing the plasmodium form of various species of malaria or the numbered column of different stages with the appropriate numbered statement.

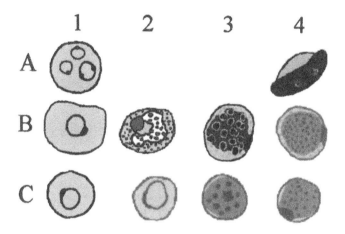

633.   Which row (A–C) illustrates the peripheral blood forms of *Plasmodium vivax*?

B is correct.
The enlarged infected erythrocytes and presence of Schuffer's dots in the trophozoite forms are characteristic of *P. vivax*.

634.   Which row (A–C) depicts *Plasmodium falciparum*?

A is correct.
The sausage-shaped gametocyte is diagnostic of the species. The absence of trophozoite and schizonts forms is because they are found in the liver and are rarely seen in peripheral blood smears.

635.   Which column (1–4) shows the sexual forms of the parasites?

Column 4 is correct.
The gametocytes require ingestion by the mosquito to complete the sexual cycle.